Drug Development and Safety

Edited by Abdur Rauf

Published in London, United Kingdom

Drug Development and Safety
http://dx.doi.org/10.5772/intechopen.111305
Edited by Abdur Rauf

Contributors
Abdur Rauf, Azim Merchant, Donia A. Al-Bastaki, Eduardo F. Mufarrege, Fazal Wahab, Florencia Rivarosa, Gladys Molina-Salinas, Habab Ali Ahmad, Hassan A. Hemeg, Joshua D. Mitchell, Kiran Seemab, Lucía C. Peña, Madeeha Shabnam, Marco Cerbón, Marina Etcheverrigaray, Muhammad Imran Khan, Muhammad Saeed Jan, Nguyen Hoang Khue Tu, Rachna Patel, Reem K. Al-Essa, Ronald Krone, Sagarkumar Kiritbhai Patel, Saima Naz, Valeria Rodríguez-Chávez, Waqas Alam, Zubair Ahmad

First published in London, United Kingdom, 2024 by IntechOpen
IntechOpen is the global imprint of INTECHOPEN LIMITED, registered in England and Wales, registration number: 11086078, 167-169 Great Portland Street, London, W1W 5PF, United Kingdom

British Library Cataloguing-in-Publication Data
A catalogue record for this book is available from the British Library

Additional hard and PDF copies can be obtained from orders@intechopen.com

Drug Development and Safety
Edited by Abdur Rauf
p. cm.

This title is part of the Pharmaceutical Science Book Series, Volume 5
Topic: Pharmacology
Series Editor: Rosario Pignatello
Topic Editor: Cristina Manuela Drăgoi
Associate Topic Editor: Alina Crenguţa Nicolae

Print ISBN 978-0-85014-231-0
Online ISBN 978-0-85014-232-7
eBook (PDF) ISBN 978-0-85014-233-4
ISSN 3033-3318

For EU product safety concerns:
IN TECH d.o.o., Prolaz Marije Krucifikse Kozulić 3, 51000 Rijeka, Croatia,
info@intechopen.com or visit our website at intechopen.com.

IntechOpen Book Series

Pharmaceutical Science

Volume 5

Aims and Scope of the Series

Pharmaceutical science focuses on the design, synthesis, formulation, targeting, distribution, safety, and efficacy of active compounds as potential therapeutics. It is a large interdisciplinary discipline that aims to integrate the basic principles of physical and organic chemistry, biochemistry, biology, and engineering to discover, develop, and characterize active compounds and to optimize the formulation and delivery of drugs in the body for offering new and improved safe and efficacious therapies against human diseases. The research areas covered by the pharmaceutical sciences range from medicinal chemistry and pharmaceutical technology to pharmacology and toxicology, which represent the preliminary phases of drug development. Medicinal chemistry involves the design and synthesis of pharmaceuticals as well as the isolation of active agents from natural sources. Computer-aided strategies are increasingly involved in this drug discovery process. Pharmaceutics is a multidisciplinary science that examines the relationships between drug formulation, delivery, distribution, and clinical outcomes. Modern clinical approaches are increasingly relying on controlled release strategies and drug delivery and targeting systems, including nanotechnological platforms (nanomedicine). Pharmacology is the science of drug action in biological systems. Pharmacologists also make drugs as tools to explore aspects of cell and tissue functions. Toxicology is the study of the adverse effects of active agents on living organisms and the ecosystem, including the prevention and amelioration of such adverse effects. This book series includes volumes on Drug Discovery, Delivery, and Pharmacology. Their overall aim is to present the latest research in the whole path of drug discovery and development from different points of view of this multidisciplinary and dynamic field.

Meet the Series Editor

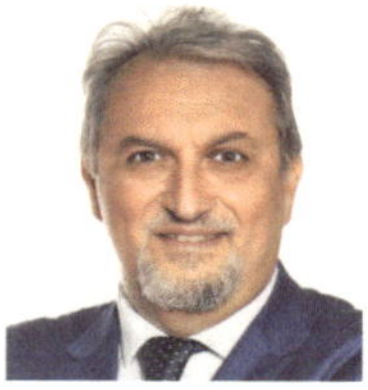

Prof. Rosario Pignatello is a Full Professor of Pharmaceutical Technology and Legislation at the University of Catania, Italy. He is the Director of the Department of Drug and Health Sciences. He has nearly 30 years of experience in the research and development of innovative formulations for the controlled release and targeting of bioactive molecules, through chemical approaches as well as nanotechnological carriers, aimed at treating different disorders. Prof. Pignatello has coauthored about 180 papers and edited a series of textbooks on biomaterials and their application in medicine. The main areas of his research are polymeric and lipid-based micro- and nanoparticles as modified drug delivery systems; vesicular nanocarriers (liposomes, micelles); lipophilic prodrugs and conjugates; synthesis and evaluation of new polymeric biomaterials for drug delivery and tissue regeneration. In particular, Prof. Pignatello works actively in the field of ocular drug delivery, leading the Research Centre for Ocular Nanotechnology, within the NANOMED Centre (Centre for Nanomedicine and Pharmaceutical Nanotechnology) at the University of Catania.

Meet the Volume Editor

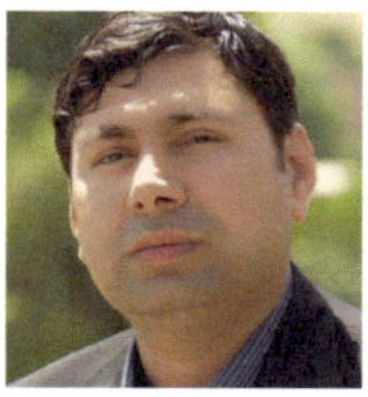

Abdur Rauf, Ph.D., is a distinguished member of the Department of Chemistry, University of Swabi, KP, Pakistan. Having earned his Ph.D. from the Institute of Chemical Sciences, University of Peshawar, Pakistan in 2015, Dr. Rauf has dedicated his career to advancing the realms of phytochemistry and pharmacology. His primary focus lies in the bio-guided isolation of new compounds for drug discovery. His scholarly contributions are remarkable, evidenced by authoring or coauthoring more than 430 research papers in esteemed peer-reviewed journals Additionally, he has edited five books and contributed thirty-nine chapters to international publications. Notably, Dr. Rauf holds one national and one international patent, with four more international patents pending, all about the discovery of novel antidiabetic drugs.

Contents

Preface

Drug development and safety are important factors in the pharmaceutical industry. The production of high-quality, effective, and safe drugs is very important for human health. The process of developing new drugs is well regulated to ensure their safety for the patients, and strict control and monitoring are maintained from the stage of development up to the clinical trials and further use on the patients.

Drug Development and Safety is a handbook for anyone who wants to get an overview of drug development's diverse facets, including drug synthesis and manufacturing, formulation and drug delivery, and drug discovery and development. How are drugs made and examined so that they are appropriate for us? In the first section, we discuss a concept known as drug repurposing, in which specialists hunt for novel methods to employ existing drugs to cure other ailments. Next, it presents a description of the rules that guarantee that drugs meet a minimum level of quality. Subsequently, we will discuss immunogenicity trials, which show how our bodies respond to new drugs. The next topic will cover cellular signaling pathways; these are important because they allow drugs to affect our body systems.

The second section of this book deals with drug delivery systems. This includes such things as controlled release systems, where medication is released into the body slowly over periods. Also included are nanotechnology-based approaches toward targeted drug delivery; for example, using nanoparticles loaded with anticancer agents for site-specific therapy. Finally, we take a look at something called bacterial minicells, which could be a new way to deliver medicines in the future.

Each chapter here is written by different scientists and specialists who are working within their scientific areas on interdisciplinary research projects. *Drug Development and Safety* aims to ensure that readers gain a thorough understanding of the importance of drug development, safety, and related topics, making it easy for chemists, pharmacists, and biologists.

Dr. Abdur Rauf, Ph.D.
Department of Chemistry,
University of Swabi,
Khyber Pakhtunkhwa, Pakistan

Section 1

Drug Development, Clinical Applications, and Regulatory Aspects

Chapter 1

Introduction to Drug Repurposing: Exploring New Applications for Existing Drugs

Zubair Ahmad, Abdur Rauf, Saima Naz and Hassan A. Hemeg

Abstract

This chapter delves into the concept of drug repurposing, which involves identifying new therapeutic applications for existing drugs. Drug repurposing offers a cost-effective and time-efficient approach to drug discovery by leveraging the knowledge and safety profiles of approved or investigational drugs. The chapter provides an overview of the principles and strategies employed in drug repurposing, including high-throughput screening, repurposing based on mechanistic insights, computational methods, and the increasing role of artificial intelligence in drug repurposing, as this is an emerging trend in the field. It explores successful case studies where repurposed drugs have shown promise in treating different diseases. Furthermore, the chapter discusses the challenges and opportunities associated with drug repurposing, including regulatory considerations and intellectual property issues. Overall, this chapter serves as a valuable resource for researchers and professionals in the field of drug development, emphasizing the potential of repurposing existing drugs to address unmet medical needs.

Keywords: drug repurposing, therapeutic applications, computational methods, high-throughput screening, efficacy

1. Introduction

Traditional drug discovery has long been a laborious and costly process, often taking years or even decades to bring a new drug to market [1]. The journey from initial target identification to clinical approval involves a high failure rate due to issues such as poor efficacy, toxicity, and unforeseen side effects [2]. These challenges have led to soaring research and development costs, making drug development increasingly unaffordable for both pharmaceutical companies and patients [3]. As a result, there is a pressing need for innovative approaches that can expedite the drug development process and increase the chances of success [4].

Drug repurposing, also known as drug repositioning or reprofiling, emerges as a promising solution to this dilemma [5]. It involves identifying new therapeutic applications for existing drugs that have already been approved for other indications or are currently undergoing investigation in clinical trials [6]. By building upon the extensive knowledge and safety profiles of these drugs, researchers can bypass several stages of preclinical testing and early clinical trials, significantly reducing both time and expenses [6].

The rationale behind drug repurposing lies in the vast reservoir of information surrounding approved drugs, including their pharmacokinetics, pharmacodynamics, and adverse event profiles [7]. These attributes offer valuable insights into how the drugs interact with the human body, their potential off-target effects, and established dosing regimens. Leveraging this information can accelerate the process of identifying new therapeutic targets and understanding the mechanisms of action, making drug repurposing a promising strategy to address unmet medical needs effectively [8].

Moreover, drug repurposing is not only advantageous for its cost-effectiveness but also for its potential to bring new treatments to patients more rapidly. It opens avenues to explore alternative therapeutic indications and expand the utility of drugs beyond their original purpose [5, 8]. As the field of drug repurposing advances, it has the potential to revolutionize the drug development landscape, offering hope for patients with limited treatment options and encouraging pharmaceutical companies to invest in areas where repurposing opportunities exist [6].

In this chapter, we delve into the principles, strategies, and success stories of drug repurposing. We explore various computational methods, high-throughput screening techniques, and mechanistic insights that drive successful drug repurposing endeavors. Additionally, we discuss the challenges and opportunities associated with this approach, ranging from regulatory considerations and intellectual property issues to funding and investment challenges. By offering a comprehensive overview of drug repurposing, this chapter aims to provide a valuable resource for researchers and professionals in the field of drug development, emphasizing the immense potential of repurposing existing drugs to address unmet medical needs.

1.1 Advantages of drug repurposing over traditional drug discovery

Drug repurposing offers several compelling advantages over the traditional drug discovery process, making it an attractive approach for addressing the challenges faced in bringing new therapeutics to market [9].

One of the most significant advantages of drug repurposing is its cost-effectiveness and time efficiency [8]. Traditional drug discovery from scratch can take up to 10–15 years and cost billions of dollars [1, 3]. In contrast, repurposing existing drugs significantly reduces the time required for drug development. By starting with compounds that have already undergone safety testing and optimization, researchers can skip the early stages of preclinical development, thereby shortening the overall timeline for getting a drug to the market. Additionally, repurposing minimizes the costs associated with preclinical and phase I clinical trials, making it a more financially viable option, especially for academic institutions and smaller pharmaceutical companies with limited resources [10, 11].

Another key advantage of drug repurposing is the access to extensive safety profiles and clinical data of already approved drugs [12]. For drugs that have been used for years or decades, there is a wealth of information available on their pharmacokinetics, pharmacodynamics, adverse events, and interactions with other drugs [13]. This knowledge significantly reduces the uncertainty associated with drug safety, streamlining the regulatory approval process. Leveraging existing clinical data also allows researchers to identify potential adverse effects and contraindications early in the drug development journey, improving patient safety and reducing the risk of unexpected side effects [14].

Repurposed drugs may also have well-established dosing regimens and formulations, which can further expedite their entry into the market [15]. By building upon this existing foundation, drug repurposing endeavors can focus more on targeted research and development, leading to quicker translation of discoveries into clinical applications. So, drug repurposing represents a compelling alternative to traditional drug discovery, offering cost-effectiveness, time efficiency, and access to well-characterized safety profiles [12]. By capitalizing on the extensive knowledge and experience of existing drugs, drug repurposing opens new opportunities to address unmet medical needs, providing hope for patients and a pathway to overcome the challenges posed by the high costs and time-intensive nature of traditional drug development [16, 17].

2. Principles of drug repurposing

The principles of drug repurposing revolve around utilizing existing drug knowledge, employing advanced data analysis tools, identifying potential therapeutic targets, and gaining mechanistic insights [18]. By harnessing the power of existing drugs and comprehensive data analyses, drug repurposing offers a strategic and efficient approach to discovering new therapeutic applications for the benefit of patients and healthcare systems alike [17, 19].

2.1 Utilizing knowledge and safety profiles of existing drugs

Existing drugs offer a wealth of valuable data that can significantly expedite the drug repurposing process [20]. These drugs have often undergone extensive preclinical and clinical testing, providing researchers with well-documented information on their pharmacokinetics, pharmacodynamics, and safety profiles [21]. By leveraging this existing knowledge, researchers can gain insights into how these drugs interact with the human body, their specific mechanisms of action, and potential off-target effects [22]. Drug repurposing efforts heavily rely on drug databases and advanced bioinformatics tools [23]. These databases aggregate information from various sources, such as clinical trials, electronic health records, and published literature, providing researchers with a comprehensive overview of drug-drug interactions, side effects, and disease associations [21, 23]. Bioinformatics tools enable researchers to identify potential therapeutic targets and predict drug-repurposing candidates by analyzing biological data, molecular structures, and computational models [24].

2.2 Identifying potential therapeutic targets for repurposing

Target identification is a crucial step in drug repurposing, aiming to uncover potential therapeutic uses for existing drugs beyond their original indications. Researchers employ various methods to identify suitable targets, focusing on disease mechanisms and common pathways [25].

Target identification methods encompass a range of approaches, including genetic studies, omics technologies (genomics, proteomics, metabolomics), and systems biology analyses [26, 27]. These methods allow researchers to unravel the molecular underpinnings of diseases, pinpoint dysfunctional genes or proteins, and identify key signaling pathways that could be modulated by repurposed drugs [28]. The success of drug repurposing often relies on understanding the underlying disease mechanisms and common molecular pathways shared by multiple diseases [28]. By identifying these shared pathways, researchers can identify drugs that have the potential to affect multiple disease conditions, broadening the scope of therapeutic applications [26].

2.3 Understanding mechanistic insights for repurposing

Mechanistic insights play a vital role in drug repurposing, guiding researchers in selecting suitable drugs and optimizing their application for new therapeutic indications [29]. Off-target effects refer to the interactions between drugs and biological targets other than the intended target. In drug repurposing, off-target effects can be both a challenge and an opportunity [30]. Understanding the off-target effects of a drug can help researchers identify additional therapeutic indications, expanding the drug's potential uses beyond its primary target [31]. Case studies are essential in illustrating the mechanistic insights gained through drug repurposing endeavors. These real-life examples highlight how drug candidates, originally developed for one condition, were successfully repurposed for other diseases based on their specific mechanisms of action and pharmacological properties [32]. These case studies provide valuable evidence and support for the feasibility and efficacy of drug repurposing.

3. Strategies for drug repurposing

3.1 Computational methods and in silico approaches

Computational methods play a crucial role in drug repurposing by enabling researchers to analyze vast databases of drugs and potential targets efficiently [33]. Virtual screening involves the use of computer algorithms to identify candidate drugs that have the potential to bind to a specific target of interest [18, 34]. Molecular docking, a common virtual screening technique, predicts the binding mode and affinity between a drug molecule and a target protein, providing insights into their interactions at the molecular level [35]. By virtually screening thousands of compounds against a target of interest, researchers can prioritize the most promising candidates for further investigation, significantly reducing the number of compounds that need to be experimentally tested [35]. Computational data analysis allows researchers to integrate information from diverse sources, such as drug databases, protein structures, and genetic data, to prioritize repurposing candidates [36]. Through machine learning algorithms and network analyses, researchers can identify potential drug-target interactions and predict the efficacy of drug candidates for different diseases [37]. Computational data-driven drug prioritization helps researchers focus their experimental efforts on the most likely candidates, leading to more efficient and targeted drug repurposing projects [38].

3.2 High-throughput screening techniques

High-throughput screening (HTS) is a powerful experimental technique that allows researchers to test thousands of compounds simultaneously for their activity against a specific biological target [39]. In drug repurposing, HTS can be employed to identify potential drug candidates that exhibit activity against a new target or disease [40]. By screening approved drugs or investigational compounds against a panel of disease-relevant targets, researchers can identify hits that show promise for further development [41].

3.3 Structure–activity relationship (SAR) analysis

Structure–activity relationship (SAR) analysis is a fundamental concept in drug discovery and development [42]. It involves studying how the chemical structure of a drug molecule influences its biological activity, such as its binding to a specific receptor or enzyme, and its subsequent pharmacological effects. By understanding SAR, researchers can gain insights into the molecular interactions that govern a drug's efficacy, potency, selectivity, and safety profile. In the context of drug repurposing, SAR analysis becomes particularly valuable [43]. Drug repurposing, also known as drug repositioning or reprofiling, refers to the process of identifying new therapeutic uses for existing drugs that were originally developed for a different medical indication [22]. This approach offers several advantages over traditional drug development, such as reduced costs, shorter development timelines, and access to a wealth of safety and pharmacokinetic data [12]. When exploring drug repurposing opportunities, researchers can leverage the knowledge gained from SAR analysis of approved drugs to identify potential candidates for new indications [44]. By identifying the critical structural features responsible for the activity against a known target, researchers can predict whether a drug may have similar interactions with a different biological target, leading to a therapeutic effect in a distinct disease context [43]. The process of SAR analysis involves synthesizing and testing structurally related analogs or derivatives of a known drug to evaluate how modifications impact its activity. These modifications can include adding or substituting functional groups, altering the core scaffold, or changing the stereochemistry [45]. Through iterative testing, researchers can determine the key structural elements responsible for a drug's activity and optimize its potency and selectivity against the desired target. Moreover, SAR analysis can help identify potential off-target effects and predict potential adverse reactions, contributing to a better understanding of a drug's overall safety profile [42]. This is especially relevant in drug repurposing, as existing drugs have already undergone significant preclinical and clinical testing, providing a wealth of safety data that can inform the decision-making process. Machine learning and computational approaches have also been employed to aid in SAR analysis [46]. By analyzing large datasets of chemical structures and biological activities, these methods can identify patterns and relationships that might not be immediately apparent through traditional experimentation.

So, SAR analysis plays a crucial role in drug repurposing efforts by providing a rational framework for identifying and optimizing drugs for new therapeutic applications. By leveraging existing knowledge of approved drugs, researchers can expedite the drug development process, potentially leading to the discovery of novel treatments for a wide range of medical conditions.

4. Examples of successful drug repurposing

Drug repurposing has proven to be a valuable strategy in medicine, providing opportunities to identify new therapeutic uses for existing drugs and expedite the development of treatments for various conditions. The examples mentioned below demonstrate how drug repurposing (**Figure 1**) can lead to significant advancements in medical care and patient outcomes across different areas of healthcare, including infectious diseases, cancer therapy, and neurological disorders.

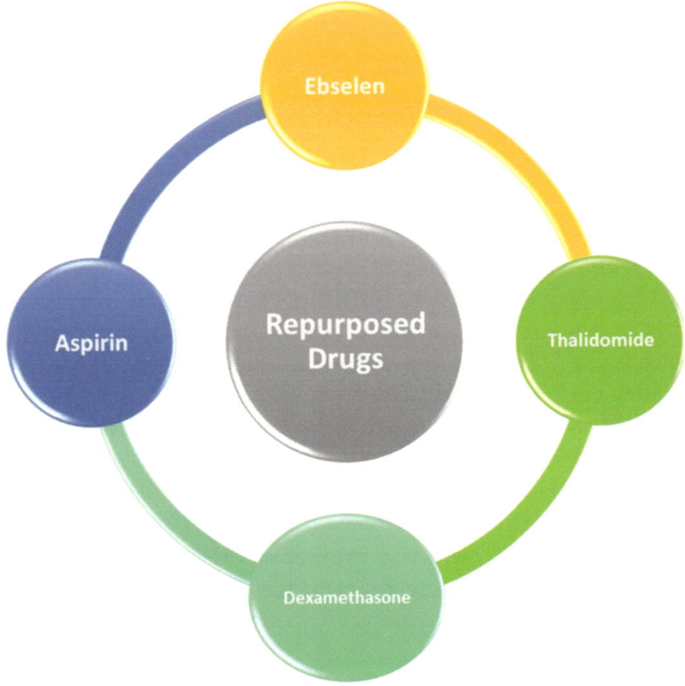

Figure 1.
List of some repurposed drugs.

4.1 Aspirin

The history of aspirin exemplifies successful drug repositioning. Originally marketed as an analgesic in 1899, it was later repurposed as an antiplatelet drug in the 1980s, leading to its widespread use for preventing cardiovascular events. Aspirin's mechanisms of action involve selective inhibition of cyclooxygenase enzymes at different doses. Ongoing research suggests a potential new repositioning of aspirin in oncology, as it has been shown to reduce the risk of developing certain cancers, including colorectal cancer, through COX-2 inhibition. However, challenges related to intellectual property issues might deter further exploration by the pharmaceutical industry in this area. Nonetheless, the history of aspirin demonstrates the importance and potential of drug repositioning in providing new therapeutic opportunities for existing medications [47].

4.2 Ebselen

Ebselen, also known as PZ-51, DR3305, and SPI-1005, is a selenorganic drug with peroxynitrite and hydroperoxide activities. It has been reported to possess cytoprotective, anti-bacterial, antioxidant, and anti-inflammatory properties, as well as acting as an apoptosis inducer and a free-radical scavenger, making it a neuroprotective agent. Ebselen has been used in the treatment of noise-induced hearing loss and bipolar mood disorder. Recent studies have shown promising antiviral activity against SARS-CoV-2, with ebselen identified as a main and papain-like protease inhibitor. It is currently undergoing phase 2 clinical trials for COVID-19 treatment.

However, further research, including *in vivo* studies and randomized clinical trials, is needed to establish its efficacy fully [48].

4.3 Thalidomide

Thalidomide, known for its tragic history of teratogenicity, was banned by the WHO in 1962 due to its harmful effects on developing fetuses. However, in 1964, Dr. Jacob Sheskin discovered its remarkable efficacy against erythema nodosum leprosum, an autoimmune complication of leprosy, which led to its repositioning by Celgene in 1998 for leprosy complications. Thalidomide's use in such cases requires stringent contraceptive measures to prevent exposure during pregnancy. In a second repositioning, thalidomide showed promise in oncology. Investigations into its teratogenic mechanism revealed its antiangiogenic activity, which inhibits blood vessel formation. This property prompted research into its potential use to block or destroy blood vessels supplying malignant tumors. In 2006, it was successfully repositioned as a first-line treatment for multiple myeloma, marking a significant advancement in its therapeutic applications [47].

4.4 Dexamethasone

Dexamethasone is a corticosteroid that was repurposed for the treatment of severe COVID-19 cases. Initially used for various inflammatory and immunosuppressive conditions, including asthma and rheumatoid arthritis, it was evaluated in clinical trials during the COVID-19 pandemic. The RECOVERY trial, conducted in the United Kingdom, demonstrated that dexamethasone reduced mortality in hospitalized COVID-19 patients requiring respiratory support, such as those on mechanical ventilation or oxygen therapy. This drug works by dampening the immune system's overreaction to the virus, particularly the cytokine storm that occurs in severe COVID-19 cases [49, 50].

5. Challenges and opportunities in drug repurposing

Drug repurposing offers significant opportunities for finding new therapeutic uses for existing drugs, but it also comes with its unique set of challenges. Despite these challenges, drug repurposing presents valuable opportunities for expanding treatment options, addressing unmet medical needs, and accelerating the drug development process. Overcoming these challenges requires innovative funding models, strong collaborations, and regulatory support to incentivize further exploration of drug repurposing potential [32].

Some of the key challenges and opportunities in drug repurposing are summarized in the inset of **Figure 2.**

5.1 Challenges

5.1.1 Limited funding for repurposing research

Drug repurposing may not attract as much funding as the development of new drugs, especially from private investors who often seek novel and exclusive products [32].

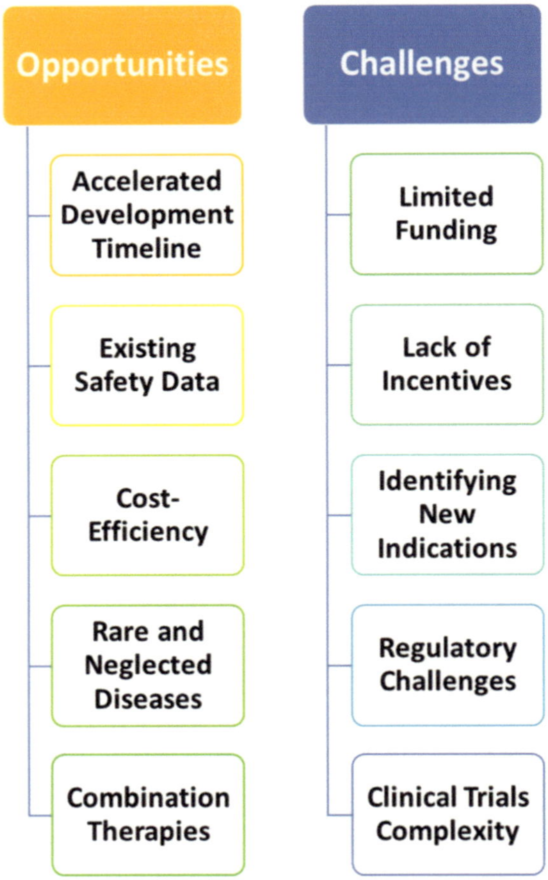

Figure 2.
Some of the key challenges and opportunities in drug repurposing.

5.1.2 Lack of incentives for pharmaceutical companies

Pharmaceutical companies may be hesitant to invest in repurposing research due to limited opportunities for patent protection and market exclusivity, which affects potential revenue streams [4].

5.1.3 Identifying new indications

Finding suitable new therapeutic uses for existing drugs requires comprehensive knowledge of the drug's pharmacology and disease mechanisms, which can be complex and time-consuming [32].

5.1.4 Regulatory challenges

Repurposing may involve using drugs for conditions outside their original approval, leading to additional regulatory requirements and uncertainties [32].

5.1.5 Clinical trials complexity

Conducting clinical trials for drug repurposing can be challenging, especially when the original drug has a well-established safety profile, and determining appropriate dosages and patient populations can be complex [4].

5.2 Opportunities

5.2.1 Accelerated development timeline

Drug repurposing can significantly reduce drug development timelines compared with starting from scratch with new chemical entities [4].

5.2.2 Existing safety data

Repurposed drugs benefit from extensive safety data gathered during their previous use, reducing the need for extensive safety testing [32].

5.2.3 Cost-efficiency

Drug repurposing can be more cost-effective than developing new drugs, as it bypasses many of the early-stage research and preclinical testing expenses [51].

5.2.4 Rare and neglected diseases

Repurposing can provide potential treatments for rare and neglected diseases, as it leverages existing drugs that might not otherwise undergo development [52].

5.2.5 Combination therapies

Repurposed drugs can be combined with existing therapies, enhancing treatment options for various medical conditions [17].

6. Conclusion

This chapter underscores the significance of drug repurposing as a pivotal strategy in contemporary drug discovery. By identifying novel therapeutic applications for established drugs, this approach offers an efficient and cost-effective route to addressing unmet medical needs. Leveraging the wealth of knowledge and safety data associated with approved or investigational drugs, drug repurposing streamlines the development process. The chapter's comprehensive exploration of principles and strategies, spanning computational methods, high-throughput screening, and mechanistic insights, illustrates the multifaceted nature of this approach. Through illuminating case studies, it becomes evident that repurposed drugs hold substantial promise in the treatment of diverse diseases. In recognizing both the challenges and opportunities inherent in drug repurposing, including regulatory and intellectual property considerations, the chapter provides a holistic view of this dynamic field. To summarize, this chapter stands as an invaluable resource, poised to guide researchers and professionals within the realm of drug development, catalyzing the realization of repurposed drugs' potential in meeting pressing medical demands.

7. Future perspective

Looking forward, the landscape of drug repurposing is poised for a series of dynamic and transformative shifts that have the potential to reshape the entire paradigm of drug development and therapeutic innovation. At the forefront of this evolution is the concept of precision medicine, which is anticipated to drive a new era of tailored repurposing strategies. With the advancement of cutting-edge technologies such as single-cell genomics and high-resolution imaging, researchers are poised to delve deeper into the intricate molecular and cellular nuances of diseases. This deeper understanding is expected to pave the way for the selection and repurposing of drugs that are precisely attuned to the unique molecular profiles of specific patient subgroups, ushering in a level of therapeutic precision previously unattainable. Moreover, the future of drug repurposing will see the convergence of multiple disciplines, with network pharmacology and the concept of synthetic lethality emerging as pivotal factors. Network pharmacology, which focuses on the intricate interactions within biological systems, promises to illuminate previously undiscovered drug targets and potential repurposing opportunities. Concurrently, the identification of synthetic lethality, where the combination of two drugs proves lethal to a particular target, could revolutionize the approach to drug repurposing by opening new avenues for the exploration of synergistic drug combinations. The scope of drug repurposing is also expected to expand beyond traditional small-molecule drugs, encompassing biologics as well. This transition is driven by the growing realization of the therapeutic potential harbored within biological drugs, including monoclonal antibodies. Repurposing biologics could unlock novel ways to address complex diseases such as cancer and autoimmune disorders, offering fresh avenues for therapeutic intervention. Crucially, the integration of artificial intelligence (AI) and machine learning into the drug repurposing landscape is anticipated to be a game-changer. These advanced algorithms are uniquely poised to rapidly sift through and analyze vast and complex datasets, predicting potential drug-disease associations, and optimizing drug combinations for enhanced synergistic effects. The resultant acceleration in data-driven insights has the potential to significantly expedite the identification of repurposed drug candidates, facilitating faster and more informed decision-making in the repurposing process. As drug repurposing continues to gain prominence on the global stage, collaboration is expected to emerge as a hallmark of future endeavors. Collaboration between researchers, pharmaceutical companies, regulatory agencies, and public health organizations is projected to accelerate the identification, validation, and deployment of repurposed drugs, particularly in response to pressing global health challenges and emergencies [53, 54].

Acknowledgements

All the authors greatly acknowledge the Department of Chemistry, University of Swabi, Khyber Pakhtunkhwa, Pakistan.

Conflict of interests

The authors declared no conflict of interest.

Author details

Zubair Ahmad[1], Abdur Rauf[1*], Saima Naz[2] and Hassan A. Hemeg[3]

1 Department of Chemistry, University of Swabi, Khyber Pakhtunkhwa, Pakistan

2 Institute of Biotechnology and Microbiology at Bacha Khan University Charsadda, Khyber Pakhtunkhwa, Pakistan

3 Department of Clinical Laboratory Sciences, College of Applied Medical Sciences, Taibah University, Al-Madinah Al-Monawra, Saudi Arabia

*Address all correspondence to: mashaljcs@yahoo.com

References

[1] Cressey DJN. Traditional drug-discovery model ripe for reform. Nature. 2011;**471**(7336):17-18

[2] Jachak SM, Saklani A. Challenges and opportunities in drug discovery from plants. Current Science. 2007;**92**(9):1251-1257

[3] Khanna I. Drug discovery in pharmaceutical industry: Productivity challenges and trends. Drug Discovery Today. 2012;**17**(19-20):1088-1102

[4] Hua Y et al. Drug repositioning: Progress and challenges in drug discovery for various diseases. European Journal of Medicinal Chemistry. 2022;**234**:114239

[5] Oprea T, Mestres J. Drug repurposing: Far beyond new targets for old drugs. The AAPS Journal. 2012;**14**:759-763

[6] Pushpakom S et al. Drug repurposing: Progress, challenges and recommendations. Nature Reviews Drug discovery. 2019;**18**(1):41-58

[7] Gns HS et al. An update on drug repurposing: Re-written saga of the drug's fate. Biomedicine & Pharmacotherapy. 2019;**110**:700-716

[8] Parvathaneni V et al. Drug repurposing: A promising tool to accelerate the drug discovery process. Drug Discovery Today. 2019;**24**(10):2076-2085

[9] Corsello SM et al. The drug repurposing hub: A next-generation drug library and information resource. Nature Medicine. 2017;**23**(4):405-408

[10] Jourdan J-P et al. Drug repositioning: A brief overview. Journal of Pharmacy and Pharmacology. 2020;**72**(9):1145-1151

[11] Mehndiratta MM et al. Drug repositioning. International Journal of Epilepsy. 2016;**3**(02):091-094

[12] Persidis A. The benefits of drug repositioning. Drug Discovery World. 2011;**12**:9-12

[13] Elder D, Tindall S. The many advantages of repurposing existing drugs. European Pharmaceutical Review. 2020;**25**(3):34-37

[14] Ashburn TT, Thor KB. Drug repositioning: Identifying and developing new uses for existing drugs. Nature Reviews Drug Discovery. 2004;**3**(8):673-683

[15] Mohammad, Jafari R et al. Drug repositioning: A review. Journal of Iranian Medical Council. 2018;**1**(1):7-10

[16] Sardana D et al. Drug repositioning for orphan diseases. Briefings in Bioinformatics. 2011;**12**(4):346-356

[17] Sun W, Sanderson PE, Zheng W. Drug combination therapy increases successful drug repositioning. Drug Discovery Today. 2016;**21**(7):1189-1195

[18] Ma D-L, Chan DS-H, Leung C-H. Drug repositioning by structure-based virtual screening. Chemical Society Reviews. 2013;**42**(5):2130-2141

[19] Padhy B, Gupta Y. Drug repositioning: Re-investigating existing drugs for new therapeutic indications. Journal of Postgraduate Medicine. 2011;**57**(2):153

[20] Tobinick EL et al. The value of drug repositioning in the current pharmaceutical market. Drug News & Perspectives. 2009;**22**(2):119-125

[21] Oprea TI, Overington JP, D.D. Technologies. Computational and practical aspects of drug repositioning. Assay and Drug Development Technologies. 2015;**13**(6):299-306

[22] Jin G, Wong ST. Toward better drug repositioning: Prioritizing and integrating existing methods into efficient pipelines. Drug Discovery Today. 2014;**19**(5):637-644

[23] Brown AS, Patel CJ. A standard database for drug repositioning. Scientific Data. 2017;**4**(1):1-7

[24] Setoain J et al. NFFinder: An online bioinformatics tool for searching similar transcriptomics experiments in the context of drug repositioning. Nucleic Acids Research. 2015;**43**(W1):W193-W199

[25] Loscalzo J. Molecular interaction networks and drug development: Novel approach to drug target identification and drug repositioning. The FASEB Journal. 2023;**37**(1)

[26] Wang W et al. Drug repositioning by integrating target information through a heterogeneous network model. Bioinformatics. 2014;**30**(20):2923-2930

[27] Hu Z-Z, et al. Omics-based molecular target and biomarker identification. Methods in Molecular Biology (Clifton, N.J.). 2011;**719**:547-571

[28] Kigondu EM et al. Pharmacologically active metabolites, combination screening and target identification-driven drug repositioning in antituberculosis drug discovery. Bioorganic & Medicinal Chemistry. 2014;**22**(16):4453-4461

[29] Padhi D, Govindaraju T. Mechanistic insights for drug repurposing and the design of hybrid drugs for Alzheimer's disease. Journal of Medicinal Chemistry. 2022;**65**(10):7088-7105

[30] Palve V et al. Turning liabilities into opportunities: Off-target based drug repurposing in cancer. In: Seminars in Cancer Biology. Elsevier; 2021

[31] Wang K et al. Prediction of drug-target interactions for drug repositioning only based on genomic expression similarity. PLoS Computational Biology. 2013;**9**(11):e1003315

[32] Novac N. Challenges and opportunities of drug repositioning. Trends in Pharmacological Sciences. 2013;**34**(5):267-272

[33] Jarada TN, Rokne JG, Alhajj R. A review of computational drug repositioning: Strategies, approaches, opportunities, challenges, and directions. Journal of Cheminformatics. 2020;**12**(1):1-23

[34] Li Z, Li X, Huang Y-Y, Wu Y, Zhou L, Liu R, et al. FEP-based screening prompts drug repositioning against COVID-19. Proceedings of the National Academy of Sciences. BioRxiv. 2020;**3**(23):004580. DOI: 10.1073/pnas.2010470117

[35] Dudley JT, Deshpande T, Butte AJ. Exploiting drug–disease relationships for computational drug repositioning. Briefings in Bioinformatics. 2011;**12**(4):303-311

[36] Xie H et al. In silico drug repositioning for the treatment of Alzheimer's disease using molecular docking and gene expression data. RSC Advances. 2016;**6**(100):98080-98090

[37] Koromina M, Pandi M-T, Patrinos GP. Rethinking drug repositioning and development with artificial intelligence, machine learning, and omics. Omics: A Journal of Integrative Biology. 2019;**23**(11):539-548

[38] Sun G et al. Drug repositioning: A bibliometric analysis. Frontiers in Pharmacology. 2022;**13**:974849

[39] Cox B et al. Application of high-throughput screening techniques to drug discovery. Progress in Medicinal Chemistry. 2000;**37**:83-134

[40] Hertzberg RP, Pope AJ. High-throughput screening: New technology for the 21st century. Current Opinion in Chemical Biology. 2000;**4**(4): 445-451

[41] Macarron R et al. Impact of high-throughput screening in biomedical research. Nature Reviews Drug Discovery. 2011;**10**(3):188-195

[42] Guha, R. On exploring structure–activity relationships. In Silico models for Drug Discovery. 2013;**993**:81-94

[43] Peltason L, Bajorath J. SAR index: Quantifying the nature of structure– activity relationships. Journal of Medicinal Chemistry. 2007;**50**(23):5571-5578

[44] Wawer M et al. Structure–activity relationship anatomy by network-like similarity graphs and local structure– activity relationship indices. Journal of Medicinal Chemistry. 2008;**51**(19):6075-6084

[45] Tong W et al. Structure-activity relationship approaches and applications. Environmental Toxicology and Chemistry: An International Journal. 2003;**22**(8):1680-1695

[46] Madugula SS et al. Molecular descriptor analysis of approved drugs using unsupervised learning for drug repurposing. Computers in Biology and Medicine. 2021;**138**:104856

[47] Jourdan J-P et al. Drug repositioning: A brief overview. Journal of Pharmacy and Pharmacology. 2020;**72**(9):1145-1151

[48] Govender K, Chuturgoon A. An overview of repurposed drugs for potential COVID-19 treatment. Antibiotics. 2022;**11**(12):1678

[49] Vaz ES et al. Drug repositioning in the COVID-19 pandemic: Fundamentals, synthetic routes, and overview of clinical studies. European Journal of Clinical Pharmacology. 2023:1-29

[50] Group, R.C. Dexamethasone in hospitalized patients with Covid-19. New England Journal of Medicine. 2021;**384**(8):693-704

[51] Turanli B, et al. Drug repositioning for effective prostate cancer treatment. Frontiers in Physiology. 2018;**9**:500

[52] Ekins S et al. In silico repositioning of approved drugs for rare and neglected diseases. Drug Discovery Today. 2011;**16**(7-8):298-310

[53] Cavalla D. Future perspectives in drug repurposing. books.rsc.org. 2022;**82**:301

[54] Wong KH, et al. Repurposing drugs for viruses and cancer: A novel drug repositioning strategy for COVID-19. Drug Repurposing for Emerging Infectious Diseases and Cancer. 2023: 423-450

Chapter 2

Building Quality into the Regulatory Review Practice for Competent Authorities

Reem K. Al-Essa and Donia A. Al-Bastaki

Abstract

The aim of this chapter is to discuss how competent authorities build quality into their assessment and registration process of medicines and to address possible challenges and opportunities for timely access to safe, effective, and high-quality medicines. Details of quality attributes which characterize the extent of scientific assessments will be the main focus. Such attributes will require solid quality management tools in place the for establishing and maintaining a proper regulatory system. Global harmonization of the regulatory review processes was achieved by the introduction of the Common Technical Document (CTD) which was developed by the International Council for Harmonization of Technical Requirements for Pharmaceuticals for Human Use (ICH) as the tool for improving the quality of the regulatory review process by standardizing the documents and specifications in the product registration dossier to minimize variations in the of assessment practices and drug approval timelines. Now, with the growing global demand for medicines and the challenges that contribute to drug shortages around the world calls for re-evaluating the impact of CTD/eCTD on the availability of medicines in a no-delay timely manner. Therefore, key quality measures must be evaluated to further harmonize and improve the speed and outcomes of the regulatory review process.

Keywords: good review practice, regulatory review, quality measures, assessment templates, common technical document

1. Introduction

Drug regulations have evolved over the last five decades in response to challenges facing the discovery development, production and distribution of pharmaceutical products. The early regulatory standards were mostly focused on guaranteeing the quality standards of the medicines, However, subsequent developments in the early 1960s led to the recognition of new standards for evaluating the safety and efficacy of new pharmaceutical products [1].

Nowadays, more challenges have occurred, mainly after the COVID-19 pandemic, which burdened the regulatory authorities around the world to meet the demand for medicines and their shortages which forced the regulators to seek other strategies to speed up the approval timelines for essential medicines without affecting their quality, safety and effectiveness. Such challenges added another impediment related to the submission of registration dossiers in the form of Common Technical Documents (CTD) and electronic Common Technical Document (eCTD) which was first adopted over two decades ago in the European Union (EU) and Japan and was the strongly recommended format for New Drug Applications (NDAs) submitted to the United States Food and Drug Administration (USFDA) to harmonize the review process around the world and to embrace the quality measures and a timely access to safe and effective medicines [2]. Therefore, building quality into the regulatory review process is important for the establishment and implementation of effective strategies to monitor the quality, minimize deficiencies and ensure reliable and timely access to safe and effective medicines [3]. However, a quality review requires regulations that are both broad and flexible to address general and specific regulatory issues [4].

In the field of pharmaceutical regulations, a pharmaceutical product can either be an investigational or a marketing application product. An investigational product refers to a therapeutic product (pharmaceutical or biological medicine), a medical device, a diagnostic, a palliative or preventive treatment (vaccine) used in clinical trial.

A marketing application is an application submitted to the regulatory authority to obtain marketing authorization for a pharmaceutical product which has not yet been approved.

The three components considered for the regulatory review process in any application are CMC, nonclinical and clinical studies. The CMC of a finished product plays an integral part in the adequate implementation of the non-clinical and clinical studies, enabling accurate analysis and association between the results obtained in each stage of the drug discovery and development process, enabling nonclinical and clinical studies and reducing a product's time to market. Efficient planning and long-range product and regulatory strategies can have lasting impacts on overall lifecycle management [5].

'Quality' is normally related to the concept of 'fitness for use' of the pharmaceutical product which meets its pre-specified quality attributes or CMC specifications [6].

Increasingly, however, 'quality' is not only being used to measure the standards of the pharmaceutical characteristics but also the drug regulatory process itself. The quality of the process, from the construction of the CTD and eCTD to the ultimate regulatory decision must also be monitored [7].

This chapter provides an overview of the measures used to build quality into the regulatory review process addressing aspects of their Good Review Practices (GRPs).

2. Defining the regulatory review quality measures

The quality measures addressed in this chapter are qualitative tools that are used to evaluate and compare the quality of the review process according to standards and benchmarks that are used to improve the competency, consistency, transparency, timeliness of the drug approval procedures [8]. The constantly changing regulatory environment requires continuous and regular optimization of efficiencies and competencies in the regulatory systems, implementing multinational endeavours to characterize assessment procedures and metrics associated with the regulatory approval systems [9].

Furthermore, solid data must always be in place identifying the milestones and overall approval times for all products from the time of submission of the registration dossier to the time of the approval of the new medicine.

Guidelines, standard operating procedures, and review templates are the building blocks for good review practices (GRP) in addition to other measures which also have an impact on the quality of the review process such as having a formal framework to apply quality decision-making practices.

Quality measures may be evaluated on a regular basis to determine their impacts on the quality and speed of the drug approval process. Timelines must be realistic, achievable and in line with the currently existing resources. Review of the human resources and the workload must always be assessed and updated according to the needs, challenges and opportunities for improving the regulatory review practices. Using the 'regulatory stop watch' to separate between the authority and the company time when setting and measuring targets is critical for both parties. The study templates should always be evaluated and improved to speed up the review process while sustaining the benefit-risk framework used for the review process adopted by the authority.

This chapter will address the general measures used to achieve quality of the review process which include tools such as communication, training and education, and transparency [8]. The chapter will also assess the drivers and barriers to achieving a quality review. An overview of the measures that determine the quality of the review process is expressed using the balance scorecard as the tool for managing the performance and outcomes of the regulatory review process [3].

3. General measures used to achieve quality

In order to build the quality of the regulatory review process, six quality measures should be considered, namely, joint and shared review (JR/SR), peer review (PR) (external and internal), assessment templates, standard operating procedures (SOPs), Good Review Practice (GRP), and a Quality Policy (QP) [3]. These are the basic measures, but other measures may be added according to the needs and challenges encountered due to the evolving regulatory environment. However, for each regulatory authority to achieve the best standards for the review practice they need to conduct a SWOT analysis to determine the strengths, weaknesses, opportunities and threats, focusing on the six quality measures stated above and pinpointing areas that require improvement in the regulatory practices.

3.1 Quality policy (QP)

QP is the overall intention and direction of an organization related to quality as formally expressed by top management. It aims to improve the performance of the reviewers, to establish whether the outcome of the review process is acceptable and whether the registration procedure fulfills the desired quality standard [3].

Therefore, in order to improve the speed and quality of the regulatory review process, consistent and continuous progress and developments musts be warranted while at the same time ensuring regular measurement and monitoring of the metrics and the outcomes of the review process addressing actions to be taken to further improve it.

3.2 Good review practice (GRP)

GRP is a documented best practice which discusses the aspects related to the process, format content and/or management of a product review. It is considered as a code for review procedures that aims to standardize and improve the overall documentation and ensure timeliness predictability, consistency and best quality reviews and review reports [8].

In order to build the quality of the review process, each authority should assess their needs and develop its own GRP for the following objectives [10]:

- The GRP is developed over time as a guideline for the best standards of review practice based on experience, and should accomplish consistency to the overall review process of new medicines.
- The GRP is developed to build quality into the regulatory review process and to improve the management tools of the review system.
- The GRP is developed to achieve better efficiency, clarity and transparency of the review process
- The GRP is developed to be adopted by the regulatory reviewers as standard procedures for the review practice which require formal training and supervised mentoring to ensure the achievement of the target metrics and outcomes.

3.3 Standard operating procedures (SOPs)

This measure is defined as the formal documents that clearly and accurately describe how an individual or organization should be performing a certain task. The purpose of a SOP is to carry out the procedures correctly and always in the same manner and should be available at the place where the work is done [3].

At regulatory authorities, reviewers use SOPs as a guidance for their scientific assessments of the registration dossiers. SOPs are revised and updated regularly according to the needs of the system and changes in the regulatory affairs and approval requirements around the world. It should always be considered as the official reference document for all reviewers, juniors or seniors, and must be readily available whenever needed. Furthermore, all appointed reviewers should be read and understand the latest version of the SOPs to achieve consistency and sustainability of the desired standards of the review practice.

3.4 Assessment report templates

Assessment templates are documents used to produce reports on the scientific review of a new active substance (NAS) for a new drug application (NDA) and an existing active substance (EAS) for an extension drug application (EDP). They provide general guidance on the evaluation of the quality, non-clinical and clinical aspects of the application [11].

Reviewers should always use an assessment template to guide their review of the registration dossier. These templates are an important quality measure that set out the content and the format of the written scientific assessment reports [8].

Assessment templates produce two types of reports:

1. Regulatory assessment reports: These are the assessment reports generated from the scientific review of the registration dossier submitted to the authority to apply for the regulatory approval of a new drug application (NDA) and an extension drug application (EDA).

2. Public assessment reports: These are published reports for every human or veterinary medicine application that has been granted or refused a marketing authorization. These types of reports follow the scientific assessment of an NDA or EDA submitted by the pharmaceutical company by the dossier registration in the format approved by the competent authority (CA) [12].

Assessment report templates coupled with SOPs form an essential component for implementing GRP.

3.5 Peer review (PR)

Peer review is an important quality measure that requires evaluation of the assessment reports by one of two persons with similar competencies to the scientific reviewer (peers). It functions as a form of self-regulation by qualified members of the regulatory profession within the review practice area. It can be implemented by establishing an internal scientific committee that evaluates the reviewer's assessment reports consisting of multidisciplinary members that evaluate each discipline of the assessment report produced by the scientific reviewer.

In addition, some CAs may carry out external peer reviews to verify that the assessment report produced by the scientific reviewer is of the desired quality and produces valid outcomes according to the data submitted in the registration dossier. This quality measure provides credibility and integrity of the review process and ensures validity and reliability of the assessment reports. However, it should be managed carefully within a reasonably monitored timelines to prevent delays in the access of medicines to patients in need. In certain cases, peer reviews may not be necessary especially for EDAs as the competency and qualification of experienced reviewers will be sufficient to grant the regulatory approval for an EAS by the registration committee that makes the final approval decision if the assessment report shows a positive outcome.

3.6 Shared/joint reviews

A shared review (SR) is the process of assigning each part or discipline within the regulatory system to the relevant expertise. For the process of medicinal product dossier review, this approach may be achieved by collaborative efforts between two or more CAs where each country is responsible for part of the registration dossier and the decision is issued to grant- or refuse to grant—the marketing approval for the product when the results are reported with recommendations to the decision-making entity (committee or person-in-charge). For example, EMA member states share expertise in the assessment of new medicinal product, relying on each other for exchange of information about the regulation of medicines [13].

Joint reviews (JRs) are usually performed jointly by several the authorities on the same application as part of a centralized regulatory system such as the one adopted by the Gulf Cooperation Council (GCC) Health Council the East African Community (EAC) [8, 14]. The Gulf States adopted the joint review initiative where the same product registration dossier is reviewed by several GCC member states. Furthermore, and the same idea have been embraced by the seven EAC countries. Therefore, a joint review is a procedure where the whole dossier is reviewed by each authority and the outcome is discussed before the decision is taken by agreement between the member states [14]. In a shared review, however, each authority takes responsibility for reviewing a separate part of the dossier.

3.7 Quality management system (QMS)

A QMS is a set of coordinated activities to direct a competent regulatory system towards improving the efficiency of its performance. It is designed and implemented to emphasize continuous improvement of the regulatory compliance and to achieve the desired outcome by making quality, safe and effective medicines readily available for patients in need [3].

QMS tools simplify the regulatory processes. They are designed to automate and integrate all quality measures and activities and to align quality across the product regulatory life cycle from the time of submission of the application for marketing approval until the time after it has been consumed by the patient where the expected clinical effect shall be met when the benefits experienced by the individual patient as well as those experienced by the society from consuming the product outweigh its individual and societal risks. QMS tools streamline processes like document control, training, risk management, Lab quality control procedures, as well as the review process to produce solid and reliable data and outcomes that improve the quality of the regulatory decision-making process.

3.8 Quality audits and feedback

Competent authorities implement several measures for continuous improvement including quality audits and feedback activities. Internal audits typically involve the organization internally auditing different units or processes. External audits are normally carried out by accredited certification bodies or external authorities, e.g., the International Organization for Standardization (ISO), the European Foundation for Quality Management (EFQM), WHO-Listed Authority (WLA). These quality audits are essential to provide the competent authority with the feedback required to improve the quality of the review process [3].

A quality audit is an essential element of Total Quality Management (TQM). It is the process of systematic and periodic on-site verification with documented examination of activities, records, practices and other components of a quality system to evaluate its degree of compliance to requirements of a standard specifications [15] such as ISO standards, Good Manufacturing Practice (GMP), Good Review Practice (GRP), Good Laboratory Practice (GLP), Good Pharmacovigilance Practice (GPvP) and Good Documentation Practice (GDocP).

In addition, it is a good practice to conduct 'post-approval' discussions with the pharmaceutical company to provide feedback on the quality of the dossier and obtain the company's comments and responses about areas of concern raised by the scientific reviewer [8]. This is a critical practice to exchange constructive feedback between the two parties for the benefit of the review outcome.

3.9 Quality assurance infrastructure

Quality is defined in a general term as 'fitness for us, focusing on compliance to regulatory requirements, conformance to obligations, and pursuit of merit and superiority'. Quality assurance (QA) is the part of the QMS focused on providing confidence that quality requirements will be fulfilled. Such confidence provided by QA is twofold: internal management of the regulatory systems, including the regulatory review process, and externally to pharmaceutical companies, external regulators, other competent authorities, certifiers and third parties [16].

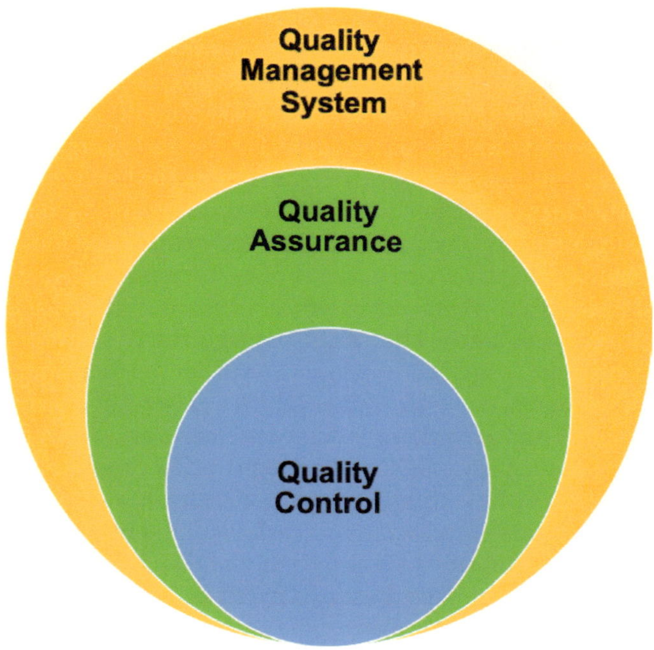

Figure 1.
Quality system, quality assurance and quality control relationships.

An alternative definition of QA is 'all the planned systematic activities implemented within the quality system that can be demonstrated to provide confidence that a product (e.g., new drug) or service (e.g., regulatory review process) will fulfil requirements for quality' [16].

Quality control (QC) is a process-oriented approach that focuses on fulfilling the quality requirement and aims to identify and rectify defects in the final product. It encompasses techniques and procedures undertaken within the quality assurance to verify that the requirements for quality have been met [17]. It involves inspecting, testing and evaluating the process or the product to ensure it meets the required standards. While QA relates to how a process is performed or how a product is made, QC is more related to the inspection/audit aspects of the quality management.

An alternate definition is 'the operational procedures and activities that fulfil the requirements of quality'.

QA infrastructure includes the QC procedures that focus on the product quality defects and require immediate actions to fulfill and maintain the quality standards. QA is part of the QMS while QC is part of the QA system (**Figure 1**).

Quality assurance should not be limited to assessment and review process but should covers all aspects of the regulatory system, medical practice and licensing.

4. Scientific committee procedure

Committees are a necessary aspect of organizations of any significant size. They formally draw together people of relevant expertise from different parts of an organization to share information and coordinate activities resulting in the widening of viewpoints and sharing of responsibilities [18]. A scientific committee involves members from multidisciplinary specialties relevant to the modules and sections presented within the registration dossier. The committee members discuss their opinions according to their expertise and share their professional insights that improve the decision-making through interactions and contribute to the committee's final recommendations and decision outcomes made by consensus. Furthermore, a scientific committee offers an opportunity for a group problem-solving and can be a medium for generating multiple ideas and by addressing a problem from various angles to come up with the best solution.

Regulatory authorities that depend on individual reviewers and decision-makers may not have the opportunity of sharing multiple viewpoints and ideas. Therefore, their decision-making process may rely on one person's thoughts and views which may lack critical insights and perspectives which may impact the final decision. The scientific committee should be the last part of the regulatory review process, being responsible for assessing the applications and generating the final approval decision. In some regulatory systems, one scientific committee exists that discusses the scientific assessment reports and generates the final decision to grant or refuse marketing authorization of the product e.g., GCC central registration committee. In other authorities, separate scientific committees exist for each area e.g., stability, quality control, GMP, Bioequivalence studies, minor variations and internal peer reviews, and external screening committee such as in UAE and Saudi Arabia [8]. All reports of the scientific committees are then discussed in the higher registration committee after the scientific committees have given their opinions and the higher registration committee makes the final approval decision [18].

4.1 Information technology (IT) infrastructure

Saudi Arabia was the first authority in the region that placed considerable efforts and resources on applying IT systems to improve the quality of the review process such as electronic tracking systems [19]. Other GCC regulatory authorities are working their ways though the system to establish an IT infrastructure that will have a positive impact on the speed, quality and efficiency of the review process. A CA seeks to implement an automated regulatory system for registration and follow-up of applications, ensuring that all the technical data (administrative, quality, nonclinical and clinical) of a pharmaceutical product are in compliance with the terms of the authorization. Furthermore, CAs approve products based on data and documents submitted at all stages of drug development from discovery to final regulatory approvals, The IT infrastructure is critical to achieve quality of the review process because it could help speed up the system by eliminating lengthy tasks and procedures for collecting, organizing and handling data from records, in addition to minimizing the human intervention in the documentation process [20]. Moreover, having an electronic system which signals delays in the review process is an important tool to control and monitor the approval timeline for pharmaceutical products [3].

Even though these facilities are available in many regulatory systems, e.g., EMA and USFDA the sophistication and the know-how of the system can differ between the various authorities [21].

4.2 Communication as a quality measure

Communication is an important aspect at any level of quality management. It plays a critical role in developing and managing any task or project. By effectively communicating information about tasks, policies, procedures, and expectations, leadership at the CA can help ensure that all regulators are on the same page and working together towards common goals for ensuring and sustaining the availability of quality, safe and effective medicines. Furthermore, communication is crucial for identifying and addressing quality issues in a timely manner.

Traditional methods are still undertaken by many CAs for communicating official policies, guidelines, memoranda and regulations to the industry using direct 'letter of request' submitted to the CA manually or electronically [19]. Some CAs (e.g., EMA, MHRA, FDA, Saudi FDA, etc) communicate official guidelines through their website which is the most convenient method for the companies.

In general, any form of communication is considered essential for the speed and quality of the regulatory review outcomes. Formal contact through scheduled meetings and official letters as well as communications through telephone conversations, SMS messages or WhatsApp messages, emails or less commonly-faxes may occur between pharmaceutical companies and authorities. The importance of effective communication between the regulators and industry cannot be overemphasized for successful and timely completion of the review process, which is particularly useful when pre-submission advice is required by the pharmaceutical company to understand the registration requirements to grant the final approval for their pharmaceutical product. Furthermore, a rational practice can be achieved when effective and transparent communication is enhanced between the pharmaceutical company and the CA. However, some authorities apply restrictions on their staff to prevent the culture of corruption from creeping into the system, and hence such authorities limit any official communication to the leadership and supervisory levels.

4.3 Training and continuous professional development

Regulatory systems cannot operate efficiently and effectively without training and comprehensive professional development programmes. Regulatory reviewers at CAs as well as the regulatory compliance personnel at the pharmaceutical industry should be equally knowledgeable and highly skilled in reviewing all parts of the registration dossier. Training could be in-house where the reviewer receives training on newly assigned duties and tasks or on changes and updates to existing ones. On the other hand, training could be received externally, either by seconding the reviewer to another authority/institution for a certain period of time to gain knowledge and insights while experiencing a different work environment, or by motivating and encouraging attendance of external professional and educational programmes and events to widen the employees' views and perspectives and expand their knowledge and skills. Ideally, after training or attending a course, the reviewer should report his/her experience or knowledge to colleagues and top managers and propose changes and improvements to existing procedures or the adoption of new practices to improve the overall performance of the reviewing staff. Proficiency test should be applied to evaluate the reviewer's competency level and to ensure that the required knowledge and skills have been achieved [8].

Training can help regulators achieve quality goals from their timely review process and efficient quality control analysis. This will reflect on the satisfaction of the patients that are able to access high quality, effective and safe medicines, as well as the satisfaction of the pharmaceutical companies that are required to fulfill the regulatory requirements efficiently and transparently.

Training is an essential quality assurance element that should be established in any CA to develop and improve processes to ensure that the final decision outcomes meet a set quality standard. Therefore, regulators should not only receive training on how to review registration dossiers or how to conduct quality control laboratory analysis, but also on quality assurance training to help all employees better understand and improve the quality of their work at all regulatory levels, policies and procedures.

4.4 Transparency as a quality measure

Transparency is an art, and leading with transparency means honoring commitments even when there are difficult decisions to be made. Regulators should be acquainted with ways to be open and honest with their colleagues and peers as well as clients, avoiding unnecessary conversations and only sticking to sharing information that best supports the future regulatory decisions that ultimately benefit the health of individuals as well as the public [22]. Transparency ensures that the review process is moving ahead towards the desired regulatory goals and producing the quality standards that are acceptable to all stakeholders. This is considered essential for establishing a relationship between the regulatory authority and other parties which is based on trust, confidence and professionalism of regulators, professionals, and the industry [8].

Transparency is an element of quality that offers no tangible incentive, but impact the CA in a positive way because it builds trust in the system, drives staff engagement and support, enhances innovation through knowledge sharing, ensures better performance, enhances collaborative attitude and encourages cooperative efforts. Furthermore, transparency builds confidence, ensures ethical conduct of the regulatory procedures and enhances the reviewer's proficiency in performing tasks and duties.

4.5 Monitoring drivers and barriers to good review practice

The most important reason for the introducing quality measures into the regulatory review process is to bring about improvement in the approval timeline while ensuring the quality, safety and effectiveness of the approved medicines. Furthermore, quality measures are adopted to minimize errors while ensuring precision, accuracy consistency and efficiency in producing the desired outcomes.

Understanding the drivers and barriers to achieving good review practice (GRP) can promote innovation and creativity while introducing new policies and procedures to help reviewers assess new medicines more efficiently and at the same time monitoring the quality of the review process and evaluating the quality of decisions made by the CA accordingly.

Drivers and barriers to the regulatory review process can be determined by three factors that contribute to its effectiveness and efficiency and can impede opportunities for making new medicines available in a timely manner. Each CA can assess its own drivers and barriers to quality based on the country's distinctive regulatory environment, its unique political situation and the governmental level of autonomy. In general, one of the major barriers identified in advanced regulatory authorities is shortages in regulatory affairs professionals and human resources when compared to projected needs for in the fields related to regulatory science [23].

5. Building quality into the regulatory review process

Having long review timelines does not necessarily imply poor performance level. Quality management tools and practices was proposed by an Empirical study which conducted in Jordan to propose organizational performance and received substantial attention in many researches [24]. Therefore, in order for the CAs to build quality into their regulatory practices, they need to create a balance between four quality assurance attributes, namely, quality measures, quality management tools, training and continuing professional development and transparent communication. This can be achieved using a balanced scorecard framework shown in **Figure 2**.

Quality measures are the first aspect in the proposed balanced scorecard framework which are considered essential practices for ensuring consistency, accuracy, competency and efficiency of the review process such as SOPs, assessment templates, GRPs, internal and external peer reviews, shared and joint reviews [18].

These can be secured if the CA has an independent QA department. Furthermore, CAs need to focus their efforts on using quality management tools more efficiently and effectively to achieve the most desired outcomes by the managerial and technical staff [25]. These activities include evaluating stakeholders' and reviewers' feedback, providing technical advice to the pharmaceutical companies on the submitted dossier, carrying out internal and external audits and establishing an electronic tracking system for monitoring the approval process (**Figure 2**).

Training and continuing professional development (CPD) programmes involve engaging expertise in association with the CAs' staff to improve the quality of their assessment through knowledge and skill transfer [26].

These programmes are critical for efficient regulatory systems because they motivate the employees to be efficient and productive. They assist them in adopting new technologies and interventions, and at the same time helps them effectively manage staff turnover and enhance creativity and innovation. This can be achieved by conducting formal training programmes for reviewers, providing placements and secondments to external CAs, attending professional development courses and post-graduate programmes and carrying out in-house and/or on-the-job training (**Figure 2**) [3]. Finally, transparency and effective communication have several advantages. They build a strong rapport

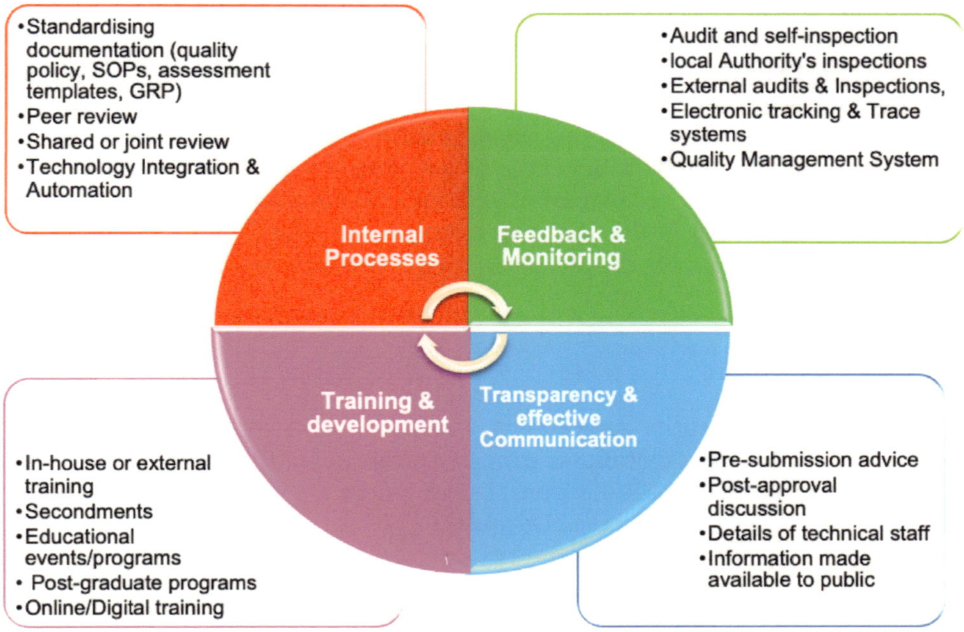

Figure 2.
Balanced scorecard framework for the types of quality measures and activities adopted by competent authorities (CAs). Source: Template adopted from [8].

between the pharmaceutical industry and regulatory authorities, enhances knowledge-based practice, supports informed decisions, and optimizes the utilization of resources, strengthens the employees' trust and job satisfaction, reduces turnover and prevents confusion, misinformation and disinformation-related critical regulatory issues. Furthermore, utilizing quality measures build trust in the system improves knowledge sharing, maintains follow-up and increases productivity and predictability of outcomes [27]. Open discussion and negotiation skills provide valuable pre-submission advice to utilize practical methods that allow better convenience and accessibility of information related to the high-quality drug approval procedure. Post-approval communications between the pharmaceutical industry and the CA is also critical to ensure sustainability of the quality, safety and effectiveness of the pharmaceutical product through the future application of improved regulatory review of future product dossiers by boosting the reviewers' knowledge and skills in the assessment process and by enhancing the confidence of the regulatory system to perform more efficiently and effectively [18].

6. Conclusion

Stringent regulatory authorities focus on the quality of the review process performed to build confidence in the drug approval system. To achieve this goal, CAs ensure the implementation of effective communication and cooperation as well as consideration of drivers for continuous advancement that fulfills the desired quality measures in the regulatory system. Therefore, CAs are required to adopt a standardized assessment template to evaluate the registration dossiers supported by SOPs to avoid lengthy timelines, to eliminate duplicate efforts and minimize variations between the assessment practices. However, to further improve the performance of good assessment practice, the authorities should apply continuous education and CPD programmes as well as adopt external quality audits from accredited certification bodies for evaluating the maturity of the regulatory system which aim at enhancing the evaluation process of the registration dossiers. Moreover, the electronic tracking system should also be adopted as a quality management tool to manage the review milestones and regulate the speed and quality of the approval system. Finally, CAs can achieve the desired quality of the review process when they thrive to improve transparency during their collaborations with the relevant stakeholders, namely, the pharmaceutical industry, healthcare professionals, patients and external peers to build trust and confidence in the pharmaceutical regulatory system.

Abbreviations

CA	Competitive authority
CMC	Chemistry, Manufacturing, Control
CPD	Continuous Professional Development
CTD	Common Technical Document
EAC	East African Community
EAS	Existing Active Substance
eCTD	Electronic Common Technical Document
EDA	Extension Drug Application
EFQM	European Foundation for Quality Management
EMA	European Medicines Agency

EU	European Union
GCC	Gulf Cooperation Council
GDocP	Good Documentation Practice
GLP	Good Laboratory Practice
GMP	Good Manufacturing Practice
GPvP	Good Pharmacovigilance Practice
GRP	Good Review Practice
ICH	International Council for Harmonization of technical Requirements for pharmaceutical Products for Human Use
ISO	International Organization for Standardization
IT	Information Technology
JR	Joint Review
KDFC	Kuwait Drug and Food Control
MHRA	Medicines and Health Regulatory Authority
NAS	New Active Substance
NDA	New Drug Application
PR	Peer Review
QA	Quality Assurance
QC	Quality Control
QMS	Quality Management System
QP	Quality Policy
Saudi FDA	Saudi Food and Drug Authority
SMS	Short Message Service
SOP	Standard Operating Procedure
SR	Shared Review
TQM	Total Quality Management
UAE	United Arab Emirates
US FDA	United Stated Food and Drug Administration

Author details

Reem K. Al-Essa[1]* and Donia A. Al-Bastaki[2]

1 Drug Inspection Administration, Drug and Food Control Sector, Ministry of Health, Kuwait

2 Head of Registration Department, Pharmaceutical and Herbal Medicines Registration and Control Administration, Drug and Food Control Sector, Ministry of Health, Kuwait

*Address all correspondence to: reem@al-essa.com

References

[1] Hill S, Johnson K. Emerging Challenges and Opportunities in Drug Registration and Regulation in Developing Countries. London: DFID Health Systems Resources Centre; 2004

[2] Jordan D. An overview of the common technical document (CTD) regulatory dossier. The European Medical Writers Association. 2014;**23**(2):101-105

[3] Al-Essa R, Salek S, Walker S. An appraisal of good regulatory review practices in the Gulf cooperation council states. Drug Information Journal. 2012;**46**:57 [Google Scholar]

[4] Brown LD, Franco LM, Rafeh N, Halzel T. Quality assurance of health care in developing countries. In: The Quality Assurance Project, U.S. Agency for International Development, Office of Health, Bureau for Science and Technology, Cooperative Agreement Number DPE-5992-A-00-0050-00 with the Center for Human Services, collaborating with Johns Hopkins University, School of Hygiene and Public Health and the Academy for Educational Development. Bethesda: Quality Assurance Project; 1998. Available from: http://www.hrhresourcecenter.org/node/796

[5] Andrade EL, Bento AF, Cavalli J, Oliveira SK, Schwanke RC, Siqueira JM, et al. Non-clinical studies in the process of new drug development - part II: Good laboratory practice, metabolism, pharmacokinetics, safety and dose translation to clinical studies. Brazilian Journal of Medical and Biological Research. 2016;**49**(12):e5646. DOI: 10.1590/1414-431X20165646

[6] Woodcock J. The concept of pharmaceutical quality. American Pharmaceutical Review. 2004;**7**(6):10-15. Available from: https://www.researchgate.net/publication/279577343_The_concept_of_pharmaceutical_quality

[7] Smith RN. Building quality measures into the regulatory review process. International Journal of Pharmaceutical Medicine. 2001;**15**:115. DOI:10.1097/00124363-200106000-00002

[8] Al-Essa R. Evaluation of the Regulation Review Processes, Quality of Decision-Making and Strategic Planning in the Gulf Cooperation Council (GCC) States. PhD Thesis. Cardiff University; 2011. Available from: https://orca.cardiff.ac.uk/id/eprint/54418/

[9] Sithole T, Mahlangu G, Salek S. Evaluation of the regulatory review process in Zimbabwe: Challenges and opportunities. Therapeutic Innovation & Regulatory Science. 2021;**55**(3):474-489

[10] FDA. Good Review Practices (GRPs); 2018. Available from: http://www.fda.gov/drugs/guidance-compliance-regulatory-information/good-review-practices-grps

[11] EMA. Assessment Templates and Guidance; 2023. Available from: https://www.ema.europa.eu/en/human-regulatory/marketing-authorisation/assessment-templates-guidance

[12] EMA. European Public Assessment Reports: Background and Context; 2023. Available from: https://www.ema.europa.eu/en/medicines/what-we-publish-when/european-public-assessment-reports-background-context

[13] EMA. The European Regulatory System for Medicines: Bringing New Safe and Effective Medicines to Patients Across the European Union; 2023.

Available from: chrome-extension://efaidnbmnnnibpcajpcglclefindmkaj/https://www.ema.europa.eu/en/documents/leaflet/european-regulatory-system-medicines_en.pdf

[14] Mashingia J, Ngum N, Ndomondo-Sigonda M, Kermad A, Bujar M, Salek S, et al. Regulatory performance of the east African community joint assessment procedure: The way forward for regulatory systems strengthening. Regulatory Toxicology and Pharmacology. May 2023;**140**:105383. DOI: 10.1016/j.yrtph.2023.105383. Epub 2023 Mar 16. PMID: 36933643

[15] Patel RB, Patel MR. Quality audit: A tool to review quality system. The Pharma Review. 2009:127-134

[16] Timmerman JG, Gardner M, Ravenscroft E. Quality Assurance. Vol. 4. UK: UN/ECE Task Force on Monitoring and Assessment. Ministry of Transport, Public Works and Water Management, RIZA Institute for Inland Water Management and Waste Water Treatment; 1996 RIZA report no.: 95.067

[17] Manghani K. Quality Assurance of Systems and Standard Operating Procedures. Perspectives in Clinical Research. 2011;**2**(1):34-37

[18] Al-Essa RK, Al-Rubaie M, Walker S, Salek S. Quality measures in the Gulf regulatory practices. In: Pharmaceutical Regulatory Environment. Cham: Adis; 2015. DOI: 10.1007/978-3-319-17590-4_4

[19] Al-Essa RK, Al-Rubaie M, Walker S, Salek S. Quality measures in the Gulf regulatory practices. In: Pharmaceutical Regulatory Environment: Challenges and Opportunities in the Gulf Region. Cham: Springer International Publishing; 2015

[20] Patil RS, Kulkarni SB, Gaikwad VL. Artificial intelligence in pharmaceutical regulatory affairs. Drug Discovery Today. 2023;**28**(9):103700. DOI: 10.1016/j.drudis.2023.103700

[21] European Medicines Agency (EMA). Guidelines on Computerised Systems and Electronic Data in Clinical Trials-Draft. Good Clinical Practice Inspectors Working Group (GCP IWG); 9 March 2023. EMA/INS/GCP/112288/2023

[22] Endres E. Taking the Lead in the Time of COVID-19 Pandemic: A Perspective from the Philippine Financial Industry. International Journal of Scientific and Research Publications (IJSRP). 2020;**10**:54-67. DOI: 10.29322/IJSRP.10.07.2020.p10307

[23] Richmond F, Church T. Talent shortage in regulatory affairs is cause for concern. Health & Medicine. 2021. Available from: http://www.researchfeatures.com

[24] Jaafreh AB, Al-abedallat AZ. The effect of quality management practices on organizational performance in Jordan: An empirical study. International Journal of Financial Research. 2013;**4**(1):93-109

[25] Mallia-Milanes A. The Development and Application of Scorecards to Assess the Quality of Regulatory Submissions and their Review. Welsh School of Pharmacy, Cardiff. Cardiff, Wales, UK: Cardiff University; 2010 [Unpublished Doctor of Philosophy]

[26] Hashan H. Evaluation of the Review Process for Marketing Pharmaceutical Products in the Gulf States and its Impact on Patients' Access to Medicines. Cardiff, Wales, UK: The Welsh School of Pharmacy, Cardiff University; 2005 [Unpublished Doctor of Philosophy]

[27] Editorial Executive Committee. Transparency-in the eye of the beholder? [editorial]. Australian Prescriber. 2005;**28**:83-84

Chapter 3

Immunogenicity Study of Biosimilar Candidates

Eduardo F. Mufarrege, Lucía C. Peña, Florencia Rivarosa and Marina Etcheverrigaray

Abstract

Therapeutic proteins can induce undesirable immune reactions in the patient and constitute a major concern as they may compromise therapy safety and efficacy. During the comparability study between a biosimilar product and the innovator, several attributes are considered. Among them, the comparative immunogenicity analysis in preclinical and clinical stages has a major relevance. In this chapter, we will describe the most used experimental platforms for biotherapeutic immunogenicity characterization. Special emphasis will be placed on *in vitro* assays for the detection of contaminants that modulate innate immune responses, as well as tools for the identification of biologic-derived T-cell epitopes. Likewise, we will also review the current trials used for the detection of host cell proteins (HCPs) and their potential impact on protein immunogenicity. Finally, we will analyze the admissibility criteria established by the Food and Drug Administration (FDA) and the European Medicines Agency (EMA), when comparing the immunogenicity of reference products and biosimilar candidates.

Keywords: immunogenicity, contaminants, T-cell epitopes, host cell proteins, *in vitro* assays, *in vivo* assays, admissibility criteria

1. Introduction

Therapeutic proteins or biotherapeutics represent a solution for the treatment of numerous human diseases [1]. Due to the complexity of these drugs and their manufacturing process, exhaustive quality control is required. Biosimilar products do not escape these control mechanisms and must comply with the eligibility criteria established by international regulatory agencies. Regarding the immunogenicity analysis of these products, the quality standards required are those achieved by the innovator product.

Protein immunogenicity represents a major concern for biologic's manufacturers due to its impact on therapy efficacy and safety. The immunogenicity of therapeutic proteins, including biosimilars, depends on several factors, including therapy-related, patient-related, and product-related issues. Here, we will focus mainly on those factors related to the biopharmaceutical product.

 IntechOpen

In humans, the immune system exhibits different checkpoints to provide cellular and molecular components that recognize and ultimately eliminate rapidly and accurately disease-causing pathogens, while avoiding damage to healthy tissue itself. This training of the immune system is widely known as immune tolerance. After the biologic is given to the patient, the therapeutic protein is screened by complex immune system surveillance processes.

For this reason, an important aspect to consider when evaluating product immunogenicity is to detect the presence of contaminants derived from the manufacturing process that can trigger innate immune responses in the patient. These entities, previously described as innate immune response modulating impurities (IIRMIs) can enhance protein immunogenicity even when present at trace levels and include microbial structures and host cell proteins (HCP) [2]. Indeed, the International Council for Harmonization (ICH) considers these impurities as critical quality attributes (CQA), that is, a product characteristic that should be within an appropriate range to ensure product quality [3].

In this chapter, we will address the state-of-the-art in current *in vitro* assays for the detection of IIRMIs. In this regard, we will establish the advantages and limitations of primary cell cultures and established cell lines designed for the specific detection of immunogenic entities.

Host cell-derived proteins (HCPs) that co-purify with the product can lead to a breakdown of immune tolerance. This unwanted immune response is triggered against the contaminating protein and, in some cases, also against the therapeutic protein [4]. While some HCPs can modulate the activity of human innate immune cells, indirectly they can also have an impact on a patient's adaptive immune responses. Once these entities bind to their receptor, they can increase the endocytic and phagocytic capacity of professional antigen-presenting cells (APCs), such as dendritic cells and macrophages, and also modulates antigen processing and peptide presentation. Consequently, these APCs can activate specific T cells, which in turn can activate B lymphocytes that differentiate into neutralizing antibodies (Nab)-producing plasma cells. In conclusion, some HCPs can act as adjuvant and modulate an undesired immune response in the patient, characterized by the generation of a pro-inflammatory scenario and subsequently by the development of antibodies against the drug and/or against the HCP. Therefore, HCPs monitoring constitutes one of the most important analytical requirements in the production of biotherapeutics.

Biotherapeutic-induced immune tolerance breakdown may also involve the adaptive immune system. As is the case with numerous proteins, biologics may contain immunogenic B- and T-cell epitopes [5–7]. As mentioned above, the presence of B-cell epitopes is closely related to the molecule's capacity to induce the production of antidrug antibodies. These antibodies can either bind to the biologic without producing a direct impact on its function or bind to the protein regions responsible for its biological effect and cause a partial or total neutralization. For this reason, Ab-mediated immune response studies in individuals treated with the biopharmaceutical have become the focus of attention during clinical trials and as a pharmacovigilance strategy [8–12].

It is widely accepted that an immune response involving the formation of high-affinity antibodies requires the collaboration of specific T cells that recognize biologic-derived epitopes [13–16]. For this reason, we will also review the most relevant *in vitro* strategies for the characterization of T-cell-mediated immune responses induced by therapeutic proteins. Specifically, we will describe the immune cell-based bioassays used to elucidate biotherapeutic-induced T-cell response profiles.

2. Detection of impurities that activate innate immune responses

Several product-specific factors can affect the immunogenic risk of biotherapeutics: product origin, primary molecular structure, posttranslational modifications, product aggregates, glycosylation/pegylation, impurities, formulation, and container closure considerations, among others [17]. In this section, we will focus on the presence of impurities in biotherapeutics and the currently available tools for their detection, and the impact prediction on product immunogenicity.

Impurities can come from the host cell or the different manufacturing process steps and can be recognized by the patient's innate immune cells, even when present at trace levels. These contaminants are widely known as innate immune response modulating impurities (IIRMIs) and include DNA, dsRNA, lipid and carbohydrate complexes, organic and inorganic components, and host cell proteins (HCPs) [2].

At present, downstream purification processes are very efficient and allow the reaching of products with high purity levels. Despite this, some contaminants can remain along with the biological product at levels not detected by the routinely used test. Moreover, *in vivo* studies in nonhuman primates showed ADA formation, when minute amounts of impurities were coadministered with a therapeutic protein [18, 19]. In addition, it was also reported that trace levels of IIRMIs could act as adjuvant and induce *in vitro* polyclonal B cell activation on murine splenocytes and consequently increase *in vivo* antibody responses [2]. Altogether, this demonstrates that very low levels of these contaminants may foster product immunogenic risk and highlights the need for tools to detect and identify IIRMIs in therapeutic products.

Currently, the analysis of IIRMIs in biologics is limited to the detection of endotoxins through the Limulus amebocyte lysate (LAL) test, PCR assays to detect host cell DNA, and ELISA-based tests for host cell proteins [20–22]. For this reason, some experimental approaches are emerging to expand the repertoire of detection of IIRMIs potentially present in biological products. Among them, the use of peripheral blood mononuclear cells (PBMCs), human and mouse monocyte/macrophage cell lines, and cell lines expressing innate immune receptors was recently proposed [23].

PBMC samples are constituted of human immune cells endowed with diverse pattern recognition receptors (PRR) capable of detecting a repertoire of IRMIIs. The results obtained by using these primary cell cultures usually mimic the *in vivo* innate immune responses observed in the clinic. The assay is based on the incubation of PBMC samples with different amounts of the tested product. Thus, whether IIRMIs are present, an increase in the expression of proinflammatory genes is observed. This experimental platform is sensitive and has a low detection limit of impurities and, as mentioned above, allows replication of the potential *in vivo* immunogenicity risk. However, some disadvantages may limit its use, such as low reproducibility, which makes it difficult to validate, limited sample availability, and safety issues associated with the handling of these cell cultures [24, 25].

Another interesting strategy involves the utilization of monocyte and macrophage cell lines. These cell lines also bear multiple innate immune receptors but without having the disadvantages associated with the use of primary cell cultures. Currently, the most widely used cell lines to detect IIRMIs in biologics are RAW 264.7 (murine macrophage); human monocytic cell line macrophage-like-MonoMac6 (MM6); and THP-1, a human monocyte cell line-derived from a patient with acute monocytic leukemia [23, 26–28]. A comprehensive study revealed that the combined use of these monocyte/macrophage cell lines allowed the recognition of a wide repertoire of IIRMIs in biotherapeutic proteins, with a detection limit similar to that achieved with PBMC samples [23].

In addition, cell engineering has also contributed to the development of strategies to specifically detect IIRMIs in biopharmaceuticals. Thus, numerous HEK293 cell lines stably expressing one or multiple PRRs and an associated reporter protein are now available [23, 29–31]. In these assays, once the cell membrane receptor is engaged by its specific ligand, these cell lines initiate a signaling cascade that culminates in the transcription activation of a reporter gene, which generates a rapidly and easily quantifiable signal.

Therefore, to carry out the adjuvant activity analysis of IIRMIs present in the biologic, it is recommended to start the study using primary cell cultures (PBMC) in combination with human and murine immune cell lines. Then, if these experimental platforms reveal the presence of IIRMIs in the product, the study can be further complemented by identifying the nature of the ligand detected through the use of HEK293 reporter cell lines.

Some reports showed the successful use of these experimental platforms for the detection and analysis of IIRMIs and their impact on biologic's safety. For instance, Haile and collaborators revealed that two IFN-β products that proved to be immunogenic in the clinic included IIRMIs in their formulation [29]. Then, the authors further explored these findings in depth and found that the increased immunogenicity was due to the presence of TLR2 and TLR4 ligands. Interestingly, none of these products evidenced the presence of endotoxins when evaluated by the LAL method. This highlights the limitations of this method for detecting low levels of this contaminant and highlights the advantages inherent in the use of cell-based assays for the detection of IIRMIs in biotherapeutics.

Additionally, a current report revealed that some excipients could mask the presence of IIRMIs. Hence, product formulation is another important issue to be considered when developing cell-based assays for IIRMIs assessment [32].

Finally, considering that comparability exercises between a reference product and the biosimilar candidate are multifactorial, these experimental platforms appear as a highly attractive alternative for measuring the immunogenicity risk of these products in the preclinical stages of development.

3. Immune responses elicited by biologic-derived T-cell epitopes

Two mechanisms culminate in the production of antidrug antibodies: a T-cell independent (Ti) and a T-cell dependent (Td) pathway. The formation of high-affinity antibodies and the generation of immune memory require the participation of T lymphocytes (TL). In addition, in the case of biotherapeutics, the Td pathway is the most likely to occur. This explains the number of studies focused on the characterization of biologic-induced T-cell responses [12–15].

Initially, dendritic cells internalize the therapeutic protein *via* vesicles. As occurs mainly with extracellular antigens, the biologic is degraded by lysosomal enzymes and the resulting peptides are presented in the context of the major histocompatibility complex class II (in humans, known as HLA-II, for human leukocyte antigen) [33]. Then, naïve TL, *via* their receptor (TCR), specifically recognize the presented peptide. From here two scenarios can be observed; if the dendritic cells express sufficient amounts of co-stimulatory molecules, the TL will be activated and differentiated toward a specific effector profile. This effector profile is driven by the dendritic cell through the cytokines secreted. Conversely, in the absence of co-stimulation, the TL becomes anergic or undergoes apoptosis [34].

B lymphocytes (BL) are also professional antigen-presenting cells (APC) and can recognize the biotherapeutic through their membrane immunoglobulin (Ig). When this occurs, internalization, processing, and antigen presentation take place similarly to as described for dendritic cells. The biologic-derived peptides are then presented to effector TL and, in the presence of appropriate co-stimulation; the TL is activated and secretes cytokines that promote BL differentiation into memory BL and ADA-producing plasma cells [35]. These antibodies can bind to the therapeutic protein (binding antibodies) without affecting its biological activity or, on the contrary, neutralizing its function (Nab). Similarly, TL also respond to this interaction producing cytokines characteristic of the acquired profile. For instance, Th1 TL secrete IFN-γ, which induces an undesired inflammatory scenario in the patient. Conversely, in the absence of specific TL responses against the biologic, the reactive BL becomes anergic or undergoes apoptosis. Therefore, the presence of biologic-derived TL epitopes not only influences the formation of high-affinity ADA, but also the generation of a pro-inflammatory response. This highlights the need for immunogenicity assays based on the detection of TL-mediated responses.

3.1 Experimental platforms for the analysis of TL-mediated immunogenicity of biosimilar products

The immune response involving high affinity and long-lasting ADA requires specific TL help. Therefore, it is recommended to perform the analysis of the immune response mediated by these cells in a preclinical stage.

Currently, there are several experimental strategies to study the TL-driven immunogenicity of biosimilar products and they are grouped into *ex vivo* and *in vivo* assays. Both experimental platforms should be carried out by including the reference product and the biosimilar candidate in the same assay, under the same experimental conditions. Thus, this head-to-head comparison will allow distinguishing differences in immunogenicity and potential risks to the patient.

3.1.1 Ex vivo assays

These experimental platforms mainly consist of collecting cells, tissues, or organs from a living organism and then performing tests based on these biological samples [36]. For instance, in assays using PBMCs, the cells can be used fresh or thawed; however, it is recommended to perform these assays from freshly extracted cells since after the freezing/thawing process the intensity of the response may be diminished. Experimental protocols may present subtle differences but in general consist of incubating PBMC cultures with the innovator product and the biosimilar candidate at a specific concentration in single or multiple antigenic stimulations. At the end of the assay, culture supernatants are extracted and various cytokines that characterize the most relevant TL response profiles are assayed [37]. A more refined experimental platform involves the prior separation of monocytes from the PBMC sample, which are then differentiated into dendritic cells (DC) using a cytokine cocktail. The DCs are then treated with the biologic and undergo a maturation process with TNF-α or LPS. Finally, the biologic-derived peptide-pulsed-DCs are co-cultured with autologous TL and the induced TL response profile is identified by cytokine profile analysis in the culture supernatant [7, 38, 39]. This experimental approach is particularly useful when the therapeutic protein has direct antiproliferative action on TL, as is the case with IFN-type I.

While the use of cell lines provides valuable, reproducible, and validatable data, primary cell cultures are still an attractive tool as they present a diversity of cellular components that correlates in composition with the *in vivo* context. For this reason, primary cell cultures derived from human peripheral blood and murine splenic cells are an interesting strategy in the preclinical stage of immunogenicity testing of innovator and biosimilar products. The most important advantages compared to established cell lines are the lower limit of detection and, as mentioned, the possibility to evaluate the immune response of multiple cellular protagonists simultaneously. The main disadvantages are the inconveniences in obtaining blood samples (availability), low reproducibility, difficulty to validate, and the safety requirements in cell culture handling [23].

3.1.2 In vivo assays

In vitro and *ex vivo* assays provide relevant information on the pattern of immune responses and allow comparison between innovative products and biosimilar candidates. However, they are still far from the *in vivo* context in clinical trials. For this reason, *in vivo* assays in model animals provide a bridge between both scenarios and allow prediction with certain accuracy of immunogenicity risks in the clinic [23]. The animal models most commonly used for immunogenicity assessments are transgenic mice tolerant to therapeutic proteins and HLA-DR mice strains [40].

3.1.2.1 Tolerant mice strains

Mice tolerant to human proteins allow mimicking human-like responses to the therapeutic version of that protein. Thus, these animal models allow identifying neo-epitopes and performing comparative immunogenicity studies of a biosimilar product and the corresponding innovator. In both cases, this animal model makes it possible to evaluate the potential breakdown of immunological tolerance toward the biologic, as a consequence of changes in the sequence, structure, and formulation of the product. The first strains developed were the human tissue plasminogen activator (htPA)-tolerant mouse [41] and the human insulin-producing animal model [42]. Both animal models proved to be valuable because of the sensitivity to detect changes of only one amino acid in the protein sequence. Later, the development of a mouse strain tolerant to human IFN-β was also useful for immunogenicity assessments of different formulations of this therapeutic protein [43].

Currently, numerous animal models tolerant to human proteins, such as growth hormone (GH) [44] and IFN-alpha [45], are available. Although these animal models are of significant utility, they have limitations associated with the murine antigenic presentation (H-2), which differs from the human system (HLA). For this reason, the use of transgenic mice expressing HLA molecules has gained great participation in preclinical immunogenicity studies.

3.1.2.2 HLA-DR-expressing transgenic mice

These mouse strains were deleted in the murine H-2 genes and instead express HLA alleles. The wide variety of HLA-DR mouse strains has allowed the extensive study of protein immunogenicity, including the identification of HLA-DR alleles with a major incidence of immunogenicity to a given biologic, as well as susceptibility or resistance to certain autoimmune diseases, infectious diseases, and vaccine efficacy [46] In addition, the utility of these transgenic mice has been confirmed by the high correlation of observed TL-mediated immune responses with results obtained later in clinical trials [47].

4. Identification and immunogenicity of HCPs in biotherapeutics

Host cell proteins (HCPs) are process-related impurities that can affect the quality and safety of biotherapeutics. Despite the efforts made during the downstream process, a little number of host endogenous proteins may co-purify with the drug substance. HCPs could be released during the fermentation process due to cell death or come from the cell lysate when the biologic is produced intracellularly. The reasons why HCPs could be present in the final product include specific or unspecific drug interaction, co-elution in chromatography steps, or due to high homology with the protein of interest [4].

4.1 Challenges and relevance of HCPs characterization

To guarantee drug purity, patient safety, and manufacturing process consistency, biotherapeutics manufacturers must demonstrate impurities and contaminants clearance. HCPs are considered a critical quality attribute [48] and regulatory guidelines [49, 50] establish that HCP levels must be monitored. Typically, 100 ppm or ng HCP/mg of therapeutic protein quantified by ELISA (see below) is the upper limit adopted in the industry [51]. However, because HCPs quantification assays for different biotherapeutics cannot be compared, it is not possible to establish a unique HCP safe threshold level.

A distinguishing feature of HCPs from other impurities is their complexity and the impossibility of predicting their profile in different product batches. Thousands of host cell proteins with high heterogeneity (molecular weight, PI, hydrophobicity, and isoforms) may accompany the biotherapeutic in the downstream process. Notably, more than 6000 HCPs have been identified in the CHO cell proteome [52] but only a few proteins are found in final products [53–55]. Surprisingly, biotherapeutics expressed at low levels as human coagulation factors may represent only 3% of the starting material for purification, being HCPs the remaining 97% [4]. As a result, HCP monitoring and clearance represent an analytical challenge for the industry.

HCP complexity also provides a spectrum of risks associated with its presence in the final product. A four-category classification of high-risk HCPs based on their impacts was proposed by the Biophorum Development Group (BPDG): (1) product quality, (2) formulation, (3) direct biological function in humans, and (4) immunogenicity [56]. They have also published a collection of high-risks CHO HCPs on mAb production and developed an online platform with updatable content (https://www.biophorum.com/host-cell-proteins/). Furthermore, an industrial examples review of problematic HCPs was reported [4]. In addition, De Zafra et al. provided a risk assessment tool for residual HCPs identified in biotherapeutics, and factors, such as HCP identity, are discussed [51]. Homolog HCP may be active in humans or induce the formation of antibodies that cross-react with endogenous proteins. In contrast, if the HCP is highly divergent to human ortholog, that is, nonmammalian hosts, such as *Escherichia coli* or yeast; they could induce a robust immune reaction in humans.

Challenges in HCP monitoring and clearance are relevant not only for innovative biotherapeutics but also for biosimilar products. Advances in proteomics provided evidence about significant changes in HCP profile according to upstream parameters (i.e., feeding, temperature, cell line, viability, and media formulation) and factors associated with the downstream process [57–59]. Consequently, it is not possible to predict biosimilar HCP content and its potential risk.

The relevance of HCP-related impact in biotherapeutics development and production highlights the necessity of analytical tools, which provide accurate and critical information on these impurities.

4.2 Analytical methodologies for HCP monitoring

Monitoring HCP in biotherapeutics development assesses product purity and process consistency [53]. In the early process, a broad population of HCPs is present, but only a small amount of residual HCP remains in the final product. Manufacturers must demonstrate the reduction of HCPs during the downstream process. Therefore, HCPs assays are employed to measure proteins present in the final product. Detection of HCP profile changes in case of process failure or modification is also desired.

4.2.1 HCP-ELISA

There is vast evidence about analytical methodologies to monitor HCP in biotherapeutics [59–62].

Currently, the anti-HCP enzyme-linked immunosorbent assay (HCP-ELISA) is the most widely used in the biopharmaceutical industry [63]. These experimental platforms are based on the use of polyclonal anti-HCP antibodies. Antibody-producing species, such as goats, sheep, or rabbits, are immunized with cell lysate or partially purified material from a null cell line fermentation. As a result, values obtained from ELISA assays are expressed as ppm of HCPs and constitute a measure of immune-equivalent nanograms of HCPs per milligram of drug substance [53]. This is a semiquantitative assay as ELISA quantification depends on the coverage and reactivity of the anti-HCP polyclonal antibodies used and the reference antigen used as standard. ELISA-based methodologies are routinely used in industry and R&D laboratories. HCP-ELISAs have several advantages, such as sensitivity (1–100 ppm) [60], selectivity, high availability, and throughput. However, no information about HCP identity or individual amount is provided. In addition, the detection of low immunogenic HCPs is compromised due to a bias in polyclonal antibody reagent development [63].

Commercial-, platform- or -product-specific HCP-ELISA could be chosen to monitor HCP levels. When using either commercial or specific ELISA assays, experiment validation is needed. In addition, coverage analysis must be done to characterize the critical reagents. Of note, differences in total HCP amounts were detected between them [53]. For instance, platform-HCP-ELISA reported 6 to 20-fold more HCP content than generic commercial ELISA. Therefore, the choice of HCP-ELISA must be carefully analyzed. In general, generic assays are widely applied in early biopharmaceutical development stages, while validated assays may be used for licensed pharmaceuticals with process-specific performance.

For antibody coverage analysis, the most common methods are Western blotting, 2D-PAGE, 2D-DIGE, and immunocapture followed by LC-MS.

4.2.2 LC-MS as an orthogonal method to HCP profiling

The lack of HCPs identity information and potential underestimation of HCP-ELISA assays bring out the relevance to apply an orthogonal approach to monitoring HCP in biopharmaceuticals. These techniques should ideally be able to detect HCPs across a wide dynamic range, follow the profile and concentration of HCPs during a bioprocess and measure small amounts of HCPs in the presence of high levels of the drug in the final product [61]. Regulators recommend the use of LC-MS as an orthogonal method [49, 50]. LC-MS has high sensitivity and allows the identification of HCPs through the downstream process [62, 64]. However, some disadvantages of this methodology include technical complexity, big data processing, and qualified staff are usually required. A recent report showed that mass spectrometry and 2D gels/PAGE for total HCP characterization and ELISAs (commercial-, process-, or platform-specific) as release tests for total HCP quantification are mainly used among 26 surveyed biopharmaceutical companies [Jonas 2021]. The authors also proposed an analytical strategy for monitoring HCPs and a workflow if high-risk HCPs were identified. In addition, HCP profiling in CHO cells [54, 56, 65, 66] and E. coli [53, 55, 67] were made taking advantage of current advances in proteomic technology.

In conclusion, knowing the exact HCP profile of a biopharmaceutical product allows the improvement of downstream processes, especially for difficult-to-remove HCPs. Additionally, analytical methods, such as specific ELISAs, may be developed to monitor the presence of high-risk HCP impurities. Proteomics studies also provide central information to implement quality-by-design (QbD) approaches to reduce HCP content in the final product [59]. Improved HCP monitoring will result in a biologic with the lowest risk related to HCP impurities, with benefits to the patient and the pharmaceutical industry [53].

Studies of the comparability of biosimilars and the innovative drug must take into consideration the monitoring and impact of the HCP profile in order to guarantee safety and product stability.

4.3 Impact of HCPs on the overall product immunogenicity

The presence of immunogenic or immunomodulatory HCPs poses a safety hazard for biopharmaceutical products. HCPs from nonhuman expression platforms can be detected as foreign to the human immune system [68]. As a result, HCPs can act as adjuvant and modulate an undesired immune response in the patient, characterized by the generation of a pro-inflammatory response and subsequently by the development of antidrug antibodies (ADAs). Additionally, cross-reactive anti-HCP antibodies may interact with endogenous human homolog proteins, neutralizing their biological activity or developing the formation of immune complexes and inducing an inflammatory scenario in the patient. ADA responses may also lead to other clinical adverse effects, such as immunotoxicity, which includes hypersensitivity reactions, cytokine release, infusion reactions, anaphylaxis, or immune complex diseases [17]. Moreover, ADAs can neutralize the biologic's efficacy and consequently affect its pharmacokinetic parameters [69].

Some examples of immunogenic HCPs are summarized in **Table 1**. Evidence linking patient safety risk to HCP exposure is limited and lacking in detail [51]. This is relevant as underestimated immune adverse effects triggered by impurities, such as

HCP identity/ information	Product/drug-related	Effect	References
E. coli ribose phosphate isomerase	Recombinant human growth hormone	Immunogenic, adjuvant	[4]
E. coli Flagellin	Recombinant human apolipoprotein A-I Milano	Adjuvant, TL5 response	[4, 70, 71]
CHO HCP	Coagulation factor IX	Immunogenic	[4]
E. coli HCPs of 20 and 30 Kda	Recombinant granulocyte-macrophage colony-stimulating factor	Immunogenic, adjuvant	[72]
CHO PBL2	Lebrikizumab	Immunogenic	[73, 74]
E. coli DnaK	scFv aggregates	adjuvant	[75]
Concentrate of *E. coli* HCPs	Ranibizumab	ocular inflammation, adjuvant	[76]

Table 1.
Summary of HCPs with reported immunogenicity.

HCPs, may result in delays and even suspension of clinical trials [70]. Moreover, even when the clinical consequences elicited by HCPs are restricted to anti-HCPs antibody formation, the economic impact of this delay in drug development may be significant. For instance, Inspiration Biopharmaceuticals had to sell IB1001's rights to another company because the clinical trial was placed on hold due to immune responses to HCPs detected in the product [4].

Semiquantitative data provided by HCP-ELISA assays is not sufficient to monitor the risk of immunogenicity in the clinic. However, a comprehensive HCP profiling, including HCP identification along with *in vitro* and *in vivo* immunogenicity assays, during product development could anticipate immunogenicity risks and thus prevent delays in clinical trials. In particular, individual risk assessments are relevant to difficult-to-remove and "repeated" HCPs, which may affect more than one biotherapeutic.

So far, only a handful of reports have addressed immunogenicity studies of individual HCPs [75, 77]. However, neither of these works addressed the immunogenicity issue by exhaustively characterizing the immune responses induced by HCPs. On the other hand, recent reports combining *in vivo* and *ex vivo* or *in vitro* assays tested biologics spiked with HCPs pools [76] or samples with more than one individual HCP [78]. As a result, this makes it difficult to correlate an observed immune response in the clinic with a specific HCP.

In addition, the advent of immune-informatics tools has allowed the development of algorithms for predicting immunogenicity risks associated with the presence of CHO cell-derived HCPs [79]. However, data obtained from this predictive analysis should be confirmed using the available experimental platforms addressed in this chapter.

Finally, it is important to note that even when most biotherapeutics contain detectable HCPs levels, the overall impact of HCPs on biologic's safety is rare. However, although there is no clear evidence of the clinical effects of HCPs, they should be monitored during the development and production of biopharmaceuticals.

5. Admissibility criteria established by regulatory agencies

The expiration of patents protecting innovative products has made possible the arrival of numerous similar biological products in the biopharmaceutical industry. However, before reaching the market, biosimilars must go through rigorous stages of supervision and meet the requirements of the regulatory agencies of the countries where the manufacturer is seeking to market its product. In this section, we will explore some of the requirements of the US and European regulatory agencies about the admissibility criteria for biosimilar products, addressing the suggestions of both institutions at the time of carrying out an application for approval.

5.1 EMA guidelines on immunogenicity assessment of biotherapeutics

The following information was obtained from "Guideline on Immunogenicity assessment of therapeutic Proteins", published by the European Medicines Agency on May 18, 2017 [80].

For nonclinical immunogenicity assessments, human and humanized therapeutic proteins will be recognized as foreign by animals; therefore, the predictability of these studies is low. In addition, nonclinical *in vitro* and *in vivo* studies to predict immunogenicity in humans are not normally required. However, according to this guideline, it is recommended to consider emerging technologies (*in vitro*, *in vivo*, and *in silico*) during development or as a first approximation of immunogenicity risk in the clinic. *In vitro* cell-based assays for testing innate and adaptive immune responses may be useful in elucidating cell-mediated responses. In addition, if the administered therapeutic protein has an endogenous counterpart, cross-reactivity reactions may also occur. In these cases, prior knowledge of the biological functions of the endogenous protein will be useful in predicting the therapy's safety risks.

Cell-mediated responses may have a major impact in those cases where unwanted effects or the biologic's pharmacodynamics may be mediated by cellular immune responses, for example, cytotoxic T-cell-mediated responses or delayed hypersensitivity reactions.

For biosimilar products, the comparative study of humoral immune responses (antibodies) as a comparability exercise is not recommended to be carried out in animals, because, as mentioned above, these studies show a low correlation with the potential immunogenicity in humans.

The analysis of antibody formation should be carried out using valid and sensitive experimental strategies. The response should therefore be studied using an experimental platform that includes a screening stage to differentiate those antibody-positive samples, a method to confirm the presence of those antibodies, and an assay to evaluate the specificity of those antibodies. Then, the guideline also recommends complementing the study by assessing the antibody-neutralizing capacity through cell-based or non-cell-based assays, depending on the biological effect exerted by the product. This experimental method should also be validated.

As mentioned above, it may also be required to determine the Ab cross-reactivity to endogenous proteins, especially in cases where the therapy safety and/or efficacy is compromised. In addition, due to the potential clinical consequences, for Ab-positive samples, the applicant should include further characterization, including the kinetic study of the Ab response, the intensity, and response duration. Also, the study should address the following aspects: Ab titer, Ab-neutralizing function, characterization of

Ab class and subclass, specificity, and affinity. In addition, other case-specific aspects may also be required.

On the other hand, other important aspects to be considered are product-related and process-related impurities, for example, HCPs. These entities can also induce the development of antibodies in the patient and should therefore be kept to the minimum level as possible. In this case, assays should be developed and validated to allow the detection of antibodies against these impurities in patient samples.

The guideline also suggests taking into consideration aspects related to the experimental platform chosen to detect antibodies in plasma and serum samples, to minimize the number of false positives cases and avoid false negatives, the epitope masking effect, matrix effect, and sample collection time, among other aspects. In addition, it also addresses aspects related to assay controls and reagents used, assay validation, and interpretation of the results.

Concerning the immunogenicity assessment of a biosimilar candidate, the EMA guideline states the following:

> *"Comparative immunogenicity studies are always needed in the development of biosimilars. Immunogenicity testing of the biosimilar and the reference product should be conducted within the biosimilar comparability exercise by using the same assay format and sampling schedule. The assays should preferably be capable of detecting antibodies against all epitopes of both biosimilar and reference molecules. If separate assays are used for the biosimilar and the reference product, this two-antigen assay approach requires careful validation to exclude any bias due to differences in sensitivity and drug tolerance. Demonstration of similar incidence of ADAs and a good concordance between the assays provides good evidence for comparable immunogenicity."*

5.2 FDA's considerations in demonstrating biosimilarity

The following is a summary of some contents extracted from the guideline for the industry: "Scientific Considerations in Demonstrating Biosimilarity to a Reference Product" published in April 2015 by the Food and Drug Administration (FDA) [81].

When demonstrating the biosimilarity of a therapeutic protein, the guideline suggests following a stepwise approach that includes, among several studies, the characterization of the clinical immunogenicity of the biosimilar candidate.

In this regard, the applicant should consider conducting a comparative analysis of the clinical immunogenicity, including the reference product and the biosimilar candidate, in an appropriate study population.

Similarly to the guidance published by EMA, the FDA guidance also indicates that immunogenicity studies conducted in animals may not predict the potential immunogenicity of therapeutic proteins in humans. However, the FDA guidance also acknowledges that antidrug antibody responses from animal studies may provide useful information on differences in immunogenicity between the reference product and the biosimilar candidate when both products are produced by different manufacturing processes.

Therefore, the clinical immunogenicity comparative study of a biosimilar product and the reference product should allow identifying potential differences as well as assessing the incidence and severity of immunogenicity events. The impact of immune responses in humans may have a direct incidence on therapy efficacy and safety. The observed effect may be variable and include alterations in the product pharmacokinetics and the development of neutralizing antibodies to both the administered product and the endogenous counterpart if present. In more severe cases, anaphylactic reactions may occur. Thus, demonstrating no clinically significant differences in the immune responses induced by the two products is key evidence for the biosimilarity of the proposed biologic.

The immunogenicity study should include aspects related to the characteristics or profile of the immune response, as well as impact analysis of the immunogenicity event, that is, impact on the biologic's efficacy. In addition, the study should include an assessment of the incidence of such immunogenicity events and the population under study.

For a premarketing study, the guideline suggests performing a head-to-head analysis in patients who have not been previously treated with the biologic (treatment-naïve patients). However, depending on the clinical experience with the tested biologic, immunogenicity assessment in a subset of patients could also be requested. This type of study allows for obtaining more substantial results as well as it is useful to determine whether the administration of the biosimilar candidate leads to a higher risk of immunogenicity. This study population should be proposed by the applicant and accepted by the agency.

A relevant aspect to take into consideration is the selection of the clinical immunogenicity endpoint. For example, antibody development and cytokine levels should be monitored taking into account immunogenicity issues that have been observed during the use of the reference product. The applicant should define the criteria for measuring the potential immune response to the product and agree with the FDA on these criteria before starting the proposed study.

In addition, another issue to be agreed upon with the agency will be the length of the study, which will depend on the following factors:

- The time of the development of humoral immunogenicity (neutralizing antibodies) and cellular immunogenicity events, as well as the possible clinical consequences, which will be reported from the sequelae observed from the use of the reference product.

- The time until the disappearance of such immunogenicity events and the sequelae observed after completion of therapy.

- The treatment duration with the product.

Regarding the characteristics of the antibody-mediated immune response, the FDA guidance states the following:

- "Titer, specificity, relevant isotype distribution, time course of development, persistence, disappearance, impact on PK, and association with clinical sequelae.

- "Neutralization of product activity: neutralizing capacity to all relevant functions (e.g., uptake and catalytic activity, neutralization for replacement enzyme therapeutics)".

The assays proposed by the applicant should include the candidate biosimilar product and the reference product. Whenever possible, both products should be tested under the same conditions, that is, in the same assay and with the same patient sample.

Finally, as mentioned above, the development and validation of these assays should be performed at the early stages of development, consulting with the agency on the sufficiency of the study before starting the immunogenicity clinical trials.

6. Conclusion

Over the last decades, therapeutic proteins have been used for the treatment of numerous chronic and non-chronic diseases, such as cancer, autoimmune diseases and disorders, diabetes, and infectious diseases. Biologic's manufacturing process is complex and therefore requires rigorous checkpoints to ensure the required quality of the final product and batch-to-batch consistency. Among the quality control requirements, product immunogenicity stands out as a critical attribute. Thus, regulatory agencies have established guidelines that allow this analysis to be approached in a careful and concerted manner. The expiration of multiple patents protecting innovative products has allowed the arrival of numerous biosimilar candidates. Similarly to reference products, biosimilars must meet different requirements during the comparability exercise. Thus, the biosimilar immunogenicity assessments should be addressed comparatively with the reference product. This study should cover aspects, such as the presence of contaminants and impurities, that induce innate immune responses and the characterization of potential adaptive immune responses in the patient. To expedite this task, different experimental platforms are currently available and allow for predicting the potential product immunogenicity before reaching clinical trials. Finally, the advent of technologies, such as single-cell sequencing, the development of micro-organoids to mimic the human immune system, and the development of *in vitro* models of human diseases, will provide more precise tools to ensure more effective and safer biologics.

Acknowledgements

This work was supported by the Consejo Nacional de Investigaciones Científícas y Técnicas (CONICET, Argentina); Agencia Nacional de Promoción Científica y Tecnológica; Universidad Nacional del Litoral. EFM and ME are members of CONICET; LCP and FR are fellows of the same institution.

Author details

Eduardo F. Mufarrege*, Lucía C. Peña, Florencia Rivarosa and Marina Etcheverrigaray
Faculty of Biochemistry and Biological Sciences, CONICET, Laboratory of Cell Culture, Biotechnological Center of Litoral—Universidad Nacional del Litoral, Santa Fe, Argentina

*Address all correspondence to: mufarrege@fbcb.unl.edu.ar

References

[1] Walsh G. Biopharmaceutical benchmarks 2014. Nature Biotechnology. 2014;**32**(10):11

[2] Verthelyi D, Wang V. Trace levels of innate immune response modulating impurities (IIRMIs) synergize to break tolerance to therapeutic proteins. PLoS One. 2010;**5**(12):e15252

[3] European Medicines Agency. ICH Guideline Q12 on Technical and Regulatory Considerations for Pharmaceutical Product Lifecycle Management [Internet]. 2020. Available from: https://www.ema.europa.eu/en/documents/scientific-guideline/ich-guideline-q12-technical-regulatory-considerations-pharmaceutical-product-lifecycle-management_en.pdf [Accessed: 2023-01-24]

[4] Vanderlaan M, Zhu-Shimoni J, Lin S, Gunawan F, Waerner T, Van Cott KE. Experience with host cell protein impurities in biopharmaceuticals. Biotechnology Progress. 2018;**34**(4):828-837

[5] Nolte KU, Günther G, von Wussow P. Epitopes recognized by neutralizing therapy-induced human anti-interferon-α antibodies are localized within the N-terminal functional domain of recombinant interferon-α2. European Journal of Immunology. 1996;**26**(9):2155-2159

[6] Bello-Rivero I, Cervantes M, Torres Y, Ferrero J, Rodríguez E, Pérez J, et al. Characterization of the immunoreactivity of anti-interferon alpha antibodies in myasthenia gravis patients. Epitope mapping. Journal of Autoimmunity. 2004;**23**(1):63-73

[7] Mufarrege EF, Giorgetti S, Etcheverrigaray M, Terry F, Martin W, De Groot AS. De-immunized and functional therapeutic (DeFT) versions of a long lasting recombinant alpha interferon for antiviral therapy. Clinical Immunology (Orlando, Fla.). 2017;**176**:31-41

[8] Deehan M, Garcês S, Kramer D, Baker MP, Rat D, Roettger Y, et al. Managing unwanted immunogenicity of biologicals. Autoimmunity Reviews. 2015;**14**(7):569-574

[9] Tatarewicz SM, Mytych DT, Manning MS, Swanson SJ, Moxness MS, Chirmule N. Strategic characterization of anti-drug antibody responses for the assessment of clinical relevance and impact. Bioanalysis. 2014;**6**(11):1509-1523

[10] Tacey R, Greway A, Smiell J, Power D, Kromminga A, Daha M, et al. The detection of anti-erythropoietin antibodies in human serum and plasma. Journal of Immunological Methods. 2003;**283**(1-2):317-329

[11] Wadhwa M, Knezevic I, Kang HN, Thorpe R. Immunogenicity assessment of biotherapeutic products: An overview of assays and their utility. Biologicals. 2015;**43**(5):298-306

[12] Wu BW, Gunn GR, Shankar G. Competitive ligand-binding assays for the detection of neutralizing antibodies. In: Tovey MG, editor. Detection and Quantification of Antibodies to Biopharmaceuticals. Hoboken, NJ, USA: John Wiley & Sons, Inc.; 2011. pp. 175-192

[13] Clark EA, Ledbetter JA. How B and T cells talk to each other. Nature. 1994;**367**(6462):425-428

[14] Klaus GGB, Choi MSK, Lam EWF, Johnson-léger C, Cliff J. CD40: A pivotal

receptor in the determination of life/death decisions in B lymphocytes. International Reviews of Immunology. 1997;**15**(1-2):5-31

[15] Koren E, De Groot AS, Jawa V, Beck KD, Boone T, Rivera D, et al. Clinical validation of the "in silico" prediction of immunogenicity of a human recombinant therapeutic protein. Clinical Immunology. 2007;**124**(1):26-32

[16] Reveille JD. The genetic basis of autoantibody production. Autoimmunity Reviews. 2006;**5**(6):389-398

[17] U.S. Department of Health and Human Services. Immunogenicity Assessment for Therapeutic Protein Products [Internet]. 2014. Available from: https://www.fda.gov/regulatory-information/search-fda-guidance-documents/immunogenicity-assessment-therapeutic-protein-products [Accessed: 2023-01-24]

[18] Kasturi SP, Skountzou I, Albrecht RA, Koutsonanos D, Hua T, Nakaya HI, et al. Programming the magnitude and persistence of antibody responses with innate immunity. Nature. 2011;**470**(7335):543-550

[19] Haile LA, Puig M, Polumuri SK, Ascher J, Verthelyi D. In vivo effect of innate immune response modulating impurities on the skin milieu using a macaque model: Impact on product immunogenicity. Journal of Pharmaceutical Sciences. 2016;**106**(3):751-760

[20] Levin J, Bang FB. Clottable protein in limulus; its localization and kinetics of its coagulation by endotoxin. Thrombosis et Diathesis Haemorrhagica. 1968;**19**(1):186-197

[21] Piehler M, Roeder R, Blessing S, Reich J. Comparison of lal and rfc assays—Participation in a proficiency test program between 2014 and 2019. Microorganisms. 2020;**8**(3):1-11

[22] Varnamkhasti FA, Kia V, Shokri R, Mehdipour Moghaddam MJ, Paryan M. Design and development of a simple method for the detection and quantification of residual host cell DNA in recombinant rotavirus vaccine. Molecular and Cellular Probes. 2021;**55**(November 2020):101674

[23] Haile LA, Puig M, Kelley-Baker L, Verthelyi D. Detection of innate immune response modulating impurities in therapeutic proteins. Allen IC, editor. PLOS ONE. 2015;**10**(4):e0125078

[24] Poole S, Thorpe R, Meager A, Gearing AJ. Assay of pyrogenic contamination in pharmaceuticals by cytokine release from monocytes. Developments in Biological Standardization. 1988;**69**:121-123

[25] Nakagawa Y, Maeda H, Murai T. Evaluation of the in vitro pyrogen test system based on proinflammatory cytokine release from human monocytes: Comparison with a human whole blood culture test system and with the rabbit pyrogen test. Clinical and Diagnostic Laboratory Immunology. 2002;**9**(3):588-597

[26] Moesby L, Jensen S, Hansen EW, Christensen JD. A comparative study of mono mac 6 cells, isolated mononuclear cells and limulus amoebocyte lysate assay in pyrogen testing. International Journal of Pharmaceutics. 1999;**191**(2):141-149

[27] Zaitseva M, Romantseva T, Blinova K, Beren J, Sirota L, Drane D, et al. Use of human MonoMac6 cells for development of in vitro assay predictive of adjuvant safety in vivo. Vaccine. 2012;**30**(32):4859-4865

[28] Mufarrege EF, Haile LA, Etcheverrigaray M, Verthelyi DI.

Multiplexed gene expression as a characterization of bioactivity for interferon Beta (IFN- β) biosimilar candidates : Impact of innate immune response modulating impurities (IIRMIs). The AAPS Journal. 2019;**21**(2):1-11

[29] Haile LA, Polumuri SK, Rao R, Kelley-baker L, Rajaiah R, Israe T, et al. Cell based assay identifies TLR2 and TLR4 stimulating impurities in interferon beta. Scientific Reports. 2017;**7**(1):10490

[30] Han Q, Bao Z, Luo MZ, Zhang JY. Assessment of innate immune response modulating impurities in glucagon for injection. PLoS One. 2022;**17**(11):e0277922

[31] Radakovics K, Battin C, Leitner J, Geiselhart S, Paster W, Stöckl J, et al. A highly sensitive cell-based TLR reporter platform for the specific detection of bacterial TLR ligands. Frontiers in Immunology. 2022;**12**(January):1-15

[32] Thacker SG, Her C, Kelley-Baker L, Ireland DDC, Manangeeswaran M, Pang ES, et al. Detection of innate immune response modulating impurities (IIRMI) in therapeutic peptides and proteins: Impact of excipients. Frontiers in Immunology. 2022;(13):970499

[33] Wieczorek M, Abualrous ET, Sticht J, Álvaro-Benito M, Stolzenberg S, Noé F, et al. Major Histocompatibility Complex (MHC) Class I and MHC Class II Proteins: Conformational plasticity in antigen presentation. Frontiers in Immunology. 2017;**8**. Available from: http://journal.frontiersin.org/article/10.3389/fimmu.2017.00292/full

[34] Sallusto F, Lanzavecchia A. The instructive role of dendritic cells on T-cell responses. Current Opinion in Immunology. 2001;**13**(3):291-298

[35] Liu W, Sohn HW, Tolar P, Pierce SK. It's all about change: The antigen-driven initiation of B-cell receptor signaling. Cold Spring Harbor Perspectives in Biology. 2010;**2**(7):a002295-a002295

[36] Lindemann M. *Ex vivo* assessment of cellular immune function—Applications in patient care and clinical studies. Tissue Antigens. 2014;**84**(5):439-449

[37] Wullner D, Zhou L, Bramhall E, Kuck A, Goletz TJ, Swanson S, et al. Considerations for optimization and validation of an in vitro PBMC derived T cell assay for immunogenicity prediction of biotherapeutics. Clinical Immunology. 2010;**137**(1):5-14

[38] Gugliotta A, Leopold MJ, Mufarrege E, Etcheverrigaray M, Kratje R, Ceaglio N, et al. Pharmacokinetics versus in vitro antiproliferative potency to design a novel hyperglycosylated hIFN-α2 biobetter. Pharmaceutical Research. 2021;**38**(1):37-50

[39] Giorgetti SI, Etcheverrigaray M, Terry F, Martin W, De Groot AS, Ceaglio N, et al. Development of highly stable and de-immunized versions of recombinant alpha interferon: Promising candidates for the treatment of chronic and emerging viral diseases. Clinical Immunology (Orlando, Fla.). 2021;**233**:108888

[40] Brinks V, Jiskoot W, Schellekens H. Immunogenicity of therapeutic proteins: The use of animal models. Pharmaceutical Research. 2011;**28**(10):2379-2385

[41] Stewart TA, Hollingshead PG, Pitts SL, Chang R, Martin LE, Oakley H. Transgenic mice as a model to test the immunogenicity of proteins altered by site-specific mutagenesis. Molecular Biology & Medicine. 1989;**6**(4):275-281

[42] Whiteley PJ, Lake JP, Selden RF, Kapp JA. Tolerance induced by physiological levels of secreted proteins in transgenic mice expressing human insulin. The Journal of Clinical Investigation. 1989;**84**(5):1550-1554

[43] Hermeling S, Jiskoot W, Crommelin D, Bornæs C, Schellekens H. Development of a transgenic mouse model immune tolerant for human interferon beta. Pharmaceutical Research. 2005;**22**(6):847-851

[44] Lee HJ, Riley G, Johnson O, Cleland JL, Kim N, Charnis M, et al. In vivo characterization of sustained-release formulations of human growth hormone. The Journal of Pharmacology and Experimental Therapeutics. 1997;**281**(3):1431-1439

[45] Braun A, Kwee L, Labow MA, Alsenz J. Protein aggregates seem to play a key role among the parameters influencing the antigenicity of interferon alpha (IFN-alpha) in normal and transgenic mice. Pharmaceutical Research. 1997;**14**(10):1472-1478

[46] Moise L, Song C, Martin WD, Tassone R, De Groot AS, Scott DW. Effect of HLA DR epitope de-immunization of factor VIII in vitro and in vivo. Clinical Immunology. 2012;**142**(3):320-331

[47] Taneja V. Cytokines pre-determined by genetic factors are involved in pathogenesis of rheumatoid arthritis. Cytokine. 2015;**75**(2):216-221

[48] European Medicines Agency. ICH Guideline Q11 on Development and Manufacture of Drug Substances (Chemical Entities and Biotechnological/Biological Entities) [Internet]. 2012. Available from: https://www.ema.europa.eu/en/documents/scientific-guideline/guideline-immunogenicity-assessment-therapeutic-proteins-revision-1_en.pdf [Accessed: 2023-01-24]

[49] European Pharmacopoeia. European Pharmacopoeia Monograph 2.6.34. Host-cell protein assays. 2017

[50] FDA. Residual host cell protein measurement in biopharmaceuticals. USP 39 Publ Gen Chapter 1132. 2016. pp. 173-82.

[51] de Zafra CLZ, Quarmby V, Francissen K, Vanderlaan M, Zhu-Shimoni J. Host cell proteins in biotechnology-derived products: A risk assessment framework. Biotechnology and Bioengineering. 2015;**112**(11):2284-2291

[52] Baycin-Hizal D, Tabb DL, Chaerkady R, Chen L, Lewis NE, Nagarajan H, et al. Proteomic analysis of Chinese hamster ovary cells. Journal of Proteome Research. 2012;**11**(11):5265-5276

[53] Pilely K, Johansen MR, Lund RR, Kofoed T, Jørgensen TK, Skriver L, et al. Monitoring process-related impurities in biologics–host cell protein analysis. Analytical and Bioanalytical Chemistry. 2022;**414**(2):747-758

[54] Gilgunn S, El-Sabbahy H, Albrecht S, Gaikwad M, Corrigan K, Deakin L, et al. Identification and tracking of problematic host cell proteins removed by a synthetic, highly functionalized nonwoven media in downstream bioprocessing of monoclonal antibodies. Journal of Chromatography. A. 2019;**1595**:28-38

[55] Wang F, Li X, Swanson M, Guetschow E, Winston M, Smith JP, et al. Holistic analytical characterization and risk assessment of residual host cell protein impurities in an active pharmaceutical ingredient synthesized by biocatalysts. Biotechnology and Bioengineering. 2022;**119**(8):2088-2104

[56] Jones M, Palackal N, Wang F, Gaza-Bulseco G, Hurkmans K, Zhao Y,

et al. "High-risk" host cell proteins (HCPs): A multi-company collaborative view. Biotechnology and Bioengineering. 2021;**118**(8):2870-2885

[57] Schenauer MR, Flynn GC, Goetze AM. Profiling the effects of process changes on residual host cell proteins in biotherapeutics by mass spectrometry. Biotechnology Progress. 2013;**29**(4):951-957

[58] Yuk IH, Nishihara J, Walker D Jr, Huang E, Gunawan F, Subramanian J, et al. More similar than different: Host cell protein production using three null CHO cell lines. Biotechnology and Bioengineering. 2015;**112**(10):2068-2083

[59] Goey CH, Alhuthali S, Kontoravdi C. Host cell protein removal from biopharmaceutical preparations: Towards the implementation of quality by design. Biotechnology Advances. 2018;**36**(4):1223-1237

[60] Tscheliessnig AL, Konrath J, Bates R, Jungbauer A. Host cell protein analysis in therapeutic protein bioprocessing—Methods and applications. Biotechnology Journal. 2013;**8**(6):655-670

[61] Bracewell DG, Francis R, Smales CM. The future of host cell protein (HCP) identification during process development and manufacturing linked to a risk-based management for their control. Biotechnology and Bioengineering. 2015;**112**(9):1727-1737

[62] Baik JY, Guo J, Lee KH. Host Cell Proteins During Biomanufacturing. In: Lee GM, Faustrup Kildegaard H, Lee SY, Nielsen J, Stephanopoulos G, editors. Cell Culture Engineering. 1st ed. Wiley: Wiley; 2019. p. 295-311.

[63] Zhu-Shimoni J, Yu C, Nishihara J, Wong RM, Gunawan F, Lin M, et al. Host cell protein testing by ELISAs and the use of orthogonal methods. Biotechnology and Bioengineering. 2014;**111**(12):2367-2379

[64] Valente KN, Levy NE, Lee KH, Lenhoff AM. Applications of proteomic methods for CHO host cell protein characterization in biopharmaceutical manufacturing. Current Opinion in Biotechnology. 2018;**53**:144-150

[65] Valente KN, Schaefer AK, Kempton HR, Lenhoff AM, Lee KH. Recovery of Chinese hamster ovary host cell proteins for proteomic analysis. Biotechnology Journal. 2014;**9**(1):87-99

[66] Molden R, Hu M, Yen ES, Saggese D, Reilly J, Mattila J, et al. Host cell protein profiling of commercial therapeutic protein drugs as a benchmark for monoclonal antibody-based therapeutic protein development. mAbs. 2021;**13**(1):1-13. DOI: 10.1080/19420862. 2021.1955811

[67] Pilely K, Nielsen SB, Draborg A, Henriksen ML, Hansen SWK, Skriver L, et al. A novel approach to evaluate ELISA antibody coverage of host cell proteins—Combining ELISA-based immunocapture and mass spectrometry. Biotechnology Progress. 2020;**36**(4):1-12

[68] Chamberlain P, Rup B. Immunogenicity risk assessment for an engineered human cytokine analogue expressed in different cell substrates. The AAPS Journal. 2020;**22**(3):1-13

[69] Swanson SJ. Immunogenicity issues in drug development. Journal of Immunotoxicology. 2006;**3**(3):165-172

[70] Reijers JAA, Malone KE, Bajramovic JJ, Verbeek R, Burggraaf J, Moerland M. Adverse immunostimulation caused by impurities: The dark side of biopharmaceuticals. British Journal of Clinical Pharmacology. 2019;**85**(7):1418-1426

[71] Huang LY, DuMontelle JL, Zolodz M, Deora A, Mozier NM, Golding B. Use of toll-like receptor assays to detect and identify microbial contaminants in biological products. Journal of Clinical Microbiology. 2009;**47**(11):3427-3434

[72] Wadhwa M, Skog AL, Bird C, Ragnhammar P, Lilljefors M, Gaines-Das R, et al. Immunogenicity of granulocyte-macrophage colony-stimulating factor (GM-CSF) products in patients undergoing combination therapy with GM-CSF. Clinical Cancer Research: An Official Journal of the American Association for Cancer Research. 1999;**5**(6):1353-1361

[73] Vanderlaan M, Sandoval W, Liu P, Nishihara J, Tsui G, Lin M, et al. A host cell protein impurity in therapeutic monoclonal antibody [internet]. BioProcess International. 2015. Available from: https://bioprocessintl.com/analytical/downstream-validation/hamster-phospholipase-b-like-2-plbl2-a-host-cell-protein-impurity-in-therapeutic-monoclonal-antibodies-derived-from-chinese-hamster-ovary-cells/ [Accessed: 2023-01-24]

[74] Fischer SK, Cheu M, Peng K, Lowe J, Araujo J, Murray E, et al. Specific immune response to phospholipase B-like 2 protein, a host cell impurity in lebrikizumab clinical material. The AAPS Journal. 2017;**19**(1):254-263

[75] Ratanji KD, Derrick JP, Kimber I, Thorpe R, Wadhwa M, Dearman RJ. Influence of *Escherichia coli* chaperone DnaK on protein immunogenicity. Immunology. 2017;**150**(3):343-355

[76] Yasuno K, Hamamura-Yasuno E, Nishimiya D, Soma M, Imaoka M, Kai K, et al. Host cell proteins induce inflammation and immunogenicity as adjuvants in an integrated analysis of in vivo and in vitro assay systems. Journal of Pharmacological and Toxicological Methods. 2020;**103**(November 2019):106694

[77] Rane SS, Dearman RJ, Kimber I, Uddin S, Bishop S, Shah M, et al. Impact of a heat shock protein impurity on the immunogenicity of biotherapeutic monoclonal antibodies. Pharmaceutical Research. 2019;**36**(4):51

[78] Jawa V, Joubert MK, Zhang Q, Deshpande M, Hapuarachchi S, Hall MP, et al. Evaluating immunogenicity risk due to host cell protein impurities in antibody-based biotherapeutics. The AAPS Journal. 2016;**18**(6):1439-1452

[79] Bailey-Kellogg C, Gutiérrez AH, Moise L, Terry F, Martin WD, De Groot AS. CHOPPI: A web tool for the analysis of immunogenicity risk from host cell proteins in CHO-based protein production. Biotechnology and Bioengineering. 2014;**111**(11):2170-2182

[80] European Medicines Agency. Guideline on Immunogenicity Assessment of Therapeutic Proteins. 2017. Available from: https://www.ema.europa.eu/en/documents/scientific-guideline/guideline-immunogenicity-assessment-therapeutic-proteins-revision-1_en.pdf [Accessed: 2023-01-24]

[81] U.S. Department of Health and Human Services F and DA. Scientific Considerations in Demonstrating Biosimilarity to a Reference Product Guidance for Industry [Internet]. 2015. Available from: https://www.fda.gov/regulatory-information/search-fda-guidance-documents/scientific-considerations-demonstrating-biosimilarity-reference-product [Accessed: 2023-01-24]

Chapter 4

Signaling Pathways in Drug Development

Habab Ali Ahmad, Kiran Seemab, Fazal Wahab and Muhammad Imran Khan

Abstract

This chapter reviews the basic principles of signal transduction and highlights its critical role in drug discovery and development. The chapter begins by explaining the concept of cellular signaling and the variety of signaling pathways that regulate critical cellular processes. It examines the key components of signaling pathways, including receptors, ligands, intercellular messengers, and effectors, and emphasizes their complex interplay. In addition, the chapter examines the role of signaling pathways as targets for drug interventions. It examines different classes of receptors, such as G protein-coupled receptors, nuclear receptors, and tyrosine kinase receptors, and discusses their activation and downstream signaling events. The various mechanisms of drug action, including agonists, antagonists, and modulators, are also studied in the context of signal transduction. In addition, the chapter highlights the importance of pathway specificity and crosstalk in drug development and highlights the challenges and opportunities associated with pharmacological modulation of pathways. It also addresses the impact of dysregulated signaling pathways in disease, and how targeted use of these pathways can lead to innovative therapeutic strategies. Finally, the chapter addresses the importance of studying signal transduction in both preclinical and clinical settings, emphasizing the need for robust and reliable tests to assess drug efficacy and safety and for effective use of therapeutics.

Keywords: signaling pathways, drug development, MAPK, PI3K-AKT, notch signaling, targeted therapy, cellular mechanisms, drug discovery, biochemical interactions, therapeutic advancements

1. Introduction

Signaling pathways play a central role in drug development and provide essential insights into the complex molecular processes underlying disease pathogenesis. Cellular signaling is a tightly regulated communication system that enables cells to respond to extracellular stimuli and maintain homeostasis. Through a series of molecular interactions, signaling pathways relay information from cell surface receptors to intracellular effectors, thereby influencing various cellular functions and behaviors. The importance of signaling pathways in drug development lies in their involvement in a variety of diseases. Dysregulation or improper activation of these signaling pathways is commonly associated with the development and progression of numerous diseases, including cancer, diabetes, cardiovascular disease, and neurological disorders [1]. Understanding the molecular intricacies of these signaling networks enables researchers to identify critical therapeutic targets and design novel drugs aimed at the precise modulation of specific signaling pathways.

Targeted therapies represent an emerging paradigm in drug development. They aim to selectively disrupt or enhance signaling pathway components. The components are causally related to disease pathogenesis [2]. Unlike traditional broad-spectrum treatments, targeted therapies offer the potential for more precise and effective interventions, while minimizing adverse effects on healthy cells and tissues. By studying the signaling pathways involved in disease, researchers can gain valuable insight into the molecular mechanisms driving pathological processes. This knowledge is crucial for identifying potential drug targets and leading to the development of novel therapeutics tailored to specific disease mechanisms [3]. Advances in signaling pathway analysis techniques have significantly accelerated drug development processes. Molecular assays, gene expression profiling, proteomics, and computational methods, such as pathway analysis and network modeling tools, provide researchers with a comprehensive understanding of complex signaling networks [4, 5]. These tools help identify key molecular players, predict drug response, and assess treatment efficacy to ultimately optimize drug development strategies.

The specific signaling pathways involved in different diseases have opened up new possibilities for targeted therapies and increased new avenue for new drug development. By identifying key components in these signaling pathways, researchers can develop more effective targeted therapies. Those key components are responsible for disease initiation or progression. The targeted drugs would specifically modulate the identified targets [6]. Targeted therapies have shown promise in treating various diseases, offering more effective and less toxic treatment options compared to traditional approaches. In summary, signaling pathways serve as crucial mediators in the development and progression of various diseases. Dysregulation of these signaling pathways can result in pathological cellular behaviors, making them attractive targets for therapeutic interventions.

Here, we will cover the basics of signaling pathways, their role in disease, and the applications of targeted therapies in drug development. Additionally, we will discuss the challenges and limitations associated with targeted pathway analysis and explore the potential of personalized medicine in the context of pathway analysis [7]. Finally, we will look at future directions in signaling pathway research and the exciting opportunities to advance drug development and revolutionize healthcare.

2. Targeted therapy

The various targeted therapies based on the modulation of signaling pathways have emerged as a promising approach in modern drug development. Unlike traditional nonspecific treatments, targeted therapies focus on specific molecular components involved in disease pathogenesis, allowing for more precise and effective interventions. Signaling pathways that control cellular responses to various external stimuli play a crucial role in disease development and progression [8]. By understanding and selectively modulating these signaling pathways, researchers can design drugs that have improved efficacy and fewer side effects. Signaling pathways are intricate networks of molecular interactions that transmit signals from cell surface receptors to intracellular effectors, ultimately affecting cellular behaviors such as proliferation, apoptosis, and differentiation. These signaling pathways are often dysregulated in numerous diseases, including cancer [9], autoimmune diseases, and metabolic disorders, making them attractive targets for therapeutic intervention [10].

This therapeutic approach involves identifying key components within these signaling pathways that drive disease progression. By specifically targeting these components, drug developers can disrupt defective signaling cascades, restore cellular homeostasis, and halt disease progression [11]. This precision in targeting offers several advantages over traditional therapies, which often target healthy cells, as well as diseased ones, leading to side effects and reduced treatment effectiveness. In cancer treatment, for example, targeted therapies have revolutionized patient care. Drugs that inhibit specific oncogenic mutations or overactive signaling pathways have shown remarkable success in curbing tumor growth and increasing survival [12]. Herceptin, an antibody-based drug that targets the HER2/neu receptor in breast cancer, is a prime example of the clinical impact of targeted therapies. By blocking overactive HER2 signaling, Herceptin has significantly improved outcomes for patients with HER2-positive breast cancer while protecting healthy cells from toxicity

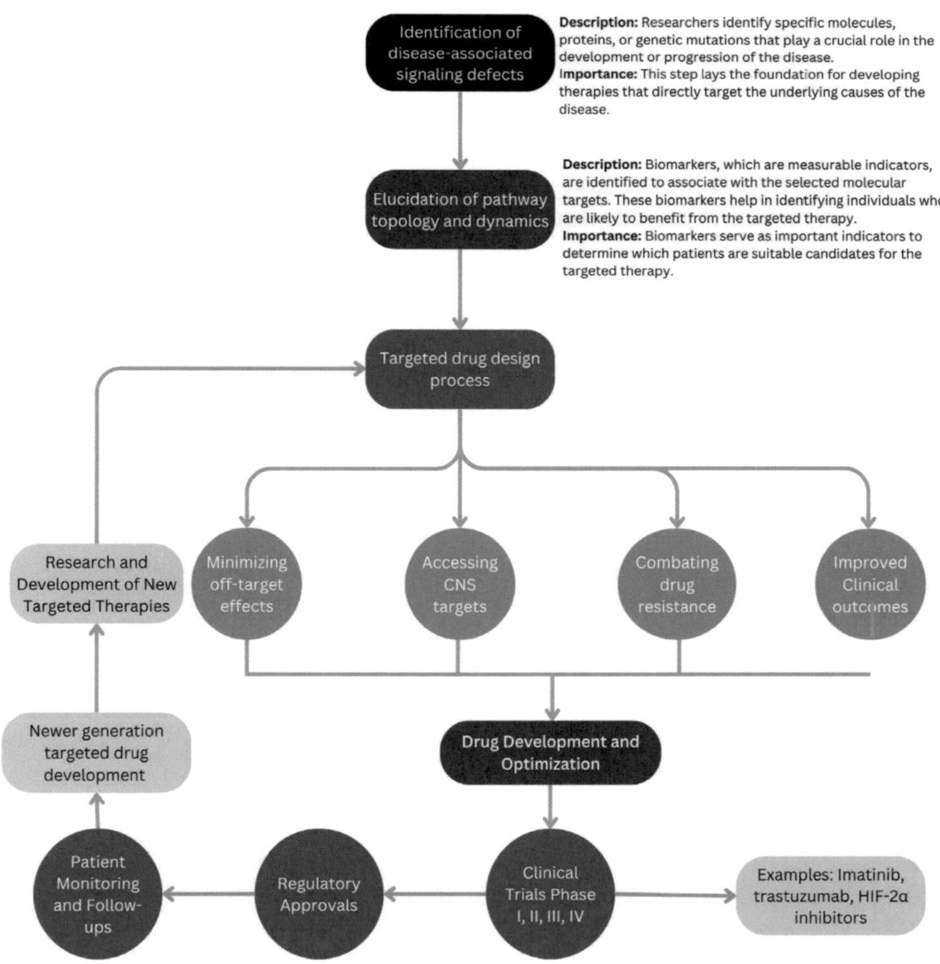

Figure 1.
Targeted therapy and drug design based on signaling pathways dysregulations.

[13]. In addition, targeted therapies have also shown promise in other disease areas. In autoimmune diseases, drugs that target specific signaling pathways, such as tumor necrosis factor (TNF) blockers in rheumatoid arthritis, have resulted in effective symptom relief and improved quality of life for patients [14]. In diabetes, drugs have been developed that modulate insulin signaling pathways to increase glucose uptake and improve glycemic level (**Figure 1**) [15].

3. Fundamentals of signaling pathways

Signaling pathways are crucial communication networks within cells that allow them to respond to external stimuli and maintain cellular homeostasis. Also, these pathways facilitate the translation of external cues into functional responses, ensuring that the cell can adapt, grow, divide, or even die in response to changing conditions. The key concepts underlying signaling pathways and their role in cellular signaling are listed below.

3.1 Components of signaling pathways

Signaling pathways have several key constituents that work in coordination to propagate and modulate signals.

Ligands: These are signaling molecules that bind to receptors. Examples include hormones, neurotransmitters, and growth factors. *Receptors:* These are proteins, often found on the cell surface, that detect ligands. Upon ligand binding, these receptors undergo a conformational change, initiating a cascade of intracellular events. *Intracellular messengers:* Once the receptor is activated, it often activates another protein inside the cell, setting off a chain reaction. These proteins can include enzymes, ion channels, and other molecules that help propagate the signal. *Effectors:* These are the final proteins in the pathway that bring about a cellular response, such as changes in gene expression, cell metabolism, or cell shape.

Cell surface receptors recognize and bind specific ligand molecules with high affinity and specificity, serving as the first step in pathway activation. Ligands themselves can have paracrine, autocrine, or endocrine activities, depending on their site of production and target cells. Kinases are a class of enzymes that add phosphate groups to proteins in a process called phosphorylation, regulating the activity of many signaling proteins. Downstream effector proteins and second messengers such as cAMP (cyclic adenosine monophosphate—second messenger that activates PKA and other effectors) amplify and transmit signals from receptors to elicit cellular outcomes such as proliferation, differentiation, growth, or apoptosis.

3.2 Types of signaling pathways

There are three major modalities of cell-cell communication mediated by signaling pathways. Firstly, receptor-mediated signaling involves ligands directly activating cell surface receptors such as receptor tyrosine kinases (RTKs: cell surface receptors with tyrosine kinase activity that propagate intracellular signals upon ligand binding) or G protein-coupled receptors (GPCRs: diverse family of cell surface receptors that activate heterotrimeric G proteins to modulate downstream signaling cascades), which, in turn, propagate intracellular signals. Secondly, intracellular signaling refers to pathways triggered within the cell, often by changes in the intracellular environment such as

Modality	Description	Examples
Receptor-mediated signaling	Ligands bind to and activate cell surface receptors, such as receptor tyrosine kinases (RTKs) and G protein-coupled receptors (GPCRs) to initiate intracellular signaling cascades.	Growth factors activating RTKs Hormones activating GPCRs
Intracellular signaling	Signaling pathways triggered inside the cell in response to changes in the intracellular environment such as fluctuations in ions, metabolites, or stress levels.	Calcium signaling in response to ion changes AMPK pathway activation by energy stress
Intercellular signaling	Cells communicate over short or long distances by secreting signaling molecules such as hormones, cytokines, or neurotransmitters into the extracellular space. These molecules then bind to receptors on neighboring (paracrine) or distant (endocrine) cells to activate signaling.	Paracrine signaling by cytokines Endocrine signaling by hormones

Table 1.
Types of cells signaling and intracellular cascade.

ion fluctuations, metabolites, or stress protein phosphorylation. Lastly, intercellular signaling enables communication between neighboring cells or distant cells through the release of signaling molecules, such as cytokines into the extracellular matrix (**Table 1**).

4. Importance of signaling pathways in drug development

4.1 Target identification

Signaling pathways provide valuable targets for drug development. By identifying key molecules within these pathways that are responsible for disease initiation or progression, researchers can develop drugs that specifically modulate these targets, leading to more effective and targeted therapies. For example, the PI3K/Akt/mTOR pathway is a central regulator of cell growth and survival. Dysregulation of this pathway is frequently observed in various cancers, leading to enhanced proliferation and survival of tumor cells. Drugs targeting PI3K or mTOR, such as idelalisib[1] and everolimus[2], have been developed as therapeutic agents for certain types of cancers.

4.2 Biomarker discovery

Signaling pathways often involve specific biomarkers that can indicate disease presence, progression, or response to treatment. By understanding the signaling events

[1] *Idelalisib* is a kinase inhibitor. Designed to target and inhibit a certain enzyme called phosphoinositide 3-kinase (PI3K). This enzyme is involved in signaling pathways that regulate cell growth, survival, and proliferation.

[2] *Everolimus* is an immunosuppressive medication that belongs to a class of drugs known as mammalian target of rapamycin (mTOR) inhibitors. It is used in transplantation and the treatment of certain types of cancer.

associated with a particular disease, researchers can identify and validate biomarkers, which can then be used to guide treatment decisions and predict patient outcomes.

For example, in breast cancer, the overexpression or amplification of the HER2/neu receptor, a component of a signaling pathway, is not only a hallmark of a specific subtype of breast cancer but also a target for therapeutic intervention using drugs, such as trastuzumab[3].

4.3 Therapeutic intervention

Personalized medicine heavily relies on the ability to intervene in specific signaling pathways based on an individual's unique molecular profile. Drugs designed to target specific molecules or mutations in signaling pathways can be tailored to each patient, maximizing therapeutic efficacy while minimizing adverse effects.

4.4 Combination therapies

Signaling pathways are complex and interconnected. Drug development in personalized medicine often involves combining targeted therapies to address multiple points within a pathway or several pathways simultaneously. Such combination therapies can enhance treatment responses and overcome drug resistance. For instance, combined inhibition of the BRAF and MEK pathways in melanoma, using drugs such as dabrafenib and trametinib, has shown improved therapeutic outcomes compared to single-agent treatments.

5. Dysregulation of signaling pathways

Dysregulation can occur in a number of ways, including:

5.1 Mutations in signaling pathway genes

Signaling pathways, integral to cellular communication, are critically reliant on the precise functionality of proteins encoded within them. When mutations arise in these genes, the proteins they produce might be altered, misfolded, or functionally aberrant, leading to disruptions in the signaling process. For instance, mutations can result in proteins that lack essential functional domains, possess unintended harmful functions, misfold to form aggregates, or alter their interaction dynamics. One of the most striking examples of the implications of such mutations is seen in the phosphoinositide 3-kinase (PI3K) pathway. This pathway, crucial in regulating cellular processes, such as growth and survival, can be severely dysregulated when the genes encoding the PI3K enzyme are mutated. Altered PI3K enzymes might continuously activate, amplify signals disproportionately, or even function without their usual triggers. Such uncontrolled activations, commonly seen in a myriad of cancers, lead to relentless cellular proliferation and survival signals, hallmark features of cancerous cells. The identification of these mutations has a threefold significance: they offer diagnostic insights, present potential therapeutic targets, and sometimes even shed light on the disease's expected progression or treatment responsiveness.

[3] *Trastuzumab* works by binding to the HER2/neu receptor on the surface of cancer cells. This binding inhibits the signaling pathways that promote the growth and division of cancer cells.

5.2 Changes in the levels of signaling pathway components

Various factors can influence the levels of signaling pathway components within cells. Among these influential factors are environmental toxins, hormones, and pharmaceutical agents. For instance, certain environmental toxins might interfere with the synthesis, degradation, or function of specific signaling proteins, leading to an accumulation or depletion of these crucial components. Similarly, hormones, which act as natural signaling molecules, can upregulate or downregulate the production of receptors or secondary messengers, thereby affecting the sensitivity and responsiveness of specific signaling pathways. Furthermore, many drugs, whether intentionally as in therapeutic agents or unintentionally as in certain contaminants, can modulate signaling pathways by altering the concentration or activity of their components. When the levels of these components are shifted, the balance and harmony of signaling processes can be disrupted. Such imbalances might not only hinder the normal functioning of cells but also pave the way for various diseases and pathological conditions. For example, an overactive signaling pathway might lead to uncontrolled cell proliferation, a hallmark of cancer, while an underactive pathway might result in cell death or impaired responses to vital environmental cues.

5.3 Abnormal activation of signaling pathways

Throughout the course of coevolutionary interactions, numerous viruses and bacteria have developed sophisticated mechanisms to exploit the intracellular signaling systems of their host organisms. These pathogens adeptly modulate the host's signaling pathways, ensuring that the cellular machinery prioritizes pathogenic replication over standard physiological functions. This strategic diversion not only undermines the host's cellular integrity but also reallocates cellular resources toward the proliferation of the invading organism. For instance, the human T-lymphotropic virus type 1 (HTLV-1) has been observed to manipulate intricate signaling networks, such as the NF-κB pathway, to enhance its own survival and propagation within the host [16].

6. Signaling pathways in disease

As researchers seek to unravel the intricate workings of cellular biology, they have become increasingly aware of the indispensable roles that dynamic signaling pathways play in orchestrating diverse physiological processes. These complex molecular circuits have evolved to allow cells to sense their environment, communicate with each other, and mount appropriate functional responses.

6.1 Cancer biosignaling

Cancer represents over 200 different diseases characterized by uncontrolled cell growth and division, driven by accumulated genetic and epigenetic alterations that promote oncogenic signaling while disabling tumor suppressive pathways. Following are the new pathways involved in cancer:

6.1.1 The Hippo pathway

The Hippo pathway is a prime example of an emerging signaling network found to be dysregulated in cancer. This pathway governs organ size control and cell proliferation through a kinase cascade that inhibits the oncogenic YAP/TAZ transcriptional coactivators when activated. However, inactivating mutations in Hippo pathway tumor suppressors, such as NF2, as well as YAP/TAZ gene amplification, have been identified across cancer types including prostate, colon, and liver cancers [17]. These alterations unleash uncontrolled growth signals that could be targeted.

6.1.2 The Wnt pathway in oncogenesis

The Wnt signaling pathway plays a vital role in fundamental processes, such as cell proliferation, migration, and differentiation, during embryogenesis and tissue homeostasis. Dysregulation of this pathway, through mutations or aberrant expression, is closely associated with cancer development and progression. The pathway can be categorized into canonical (β-catenin-dependent) and noncanonical (β-catenin-independent) pathways. Mutations in key components, such as the APC gene or β-catenin, can lead to constitutive activation of the pathway and uncontrolled cellular proliferation, particularly in colorectal carcinomas. Noncanonical pathways influence cell polarity, migration, and calcium homeostasis, with complex roles in oncogenesis dependent on the tumor microenvironment. Interactions between canonical and noncanonical pathways further modulate tumor dynamics. Therapeutically, the Wnt pathway is an attractive target, with molecules, such as tankyrase inhibitors and porcupine inhibitors, showing promise in preclinical models.

6.1.3 The Notch pathway

The Notch pathway also plays crucial roles in development and cell fate decisions. Notch is inappropriately switched on in many hematological and solid malignancies *via* overexpression, gene amplification, or loss of regulatory microRNAs. Inhibiting novel rogue pathways such as these, either alone or in combination with conventional targeted therapies, offers new therapeutic inroads against cancer (**Figure 2**).

The signaling landscape in cancer continues to grow more complex as research unravels additional contributing pathways. Mapping out these intricate molecular networks through multi-omics profiling and bioinformatics will be key to matching specific pathway dependencies to personalized targeted treatments. Somatic mutations affecting key signaling proteins, such as receptor tyrosine kinases, RAS small GTPases, and PI3K enzymes, lead to activation of pro-growth and survival cascades such as MAPK (mitogen-activated protein kinase—serine/threonine kinase signaling cascade (ERK, JNK, p38) involved in cell proliferation, differentiation, survival), PI3K/AKT (phosphatidylinositol 3-kinase—lipid kinase that generates second messengers to activate AKT and other pathways), and JAK/STAT (signal transducer and activator of transcription—transcription factors activated by cytokine receptors to regulate immune responses, proliferation, differentiation). Conversely, mutations causing loss of function in tumor suppressor genes such as PTEN, APC, and RB eliminate negative regulation, allowing unrestrained oncogenic signaling.

6.2 Diabetes and biosignaling

Diabetes mellitus comprises a group of metabolic disorders characterized by chronic hyperglycemia, resulting from defects in insulin secretion by pancreatic beta cells and/or insulin sensitivity in target tissues. In type 1 diabetes, autoimmune

DOI: http://dx.doi.org/10.5772/intechopen.114041

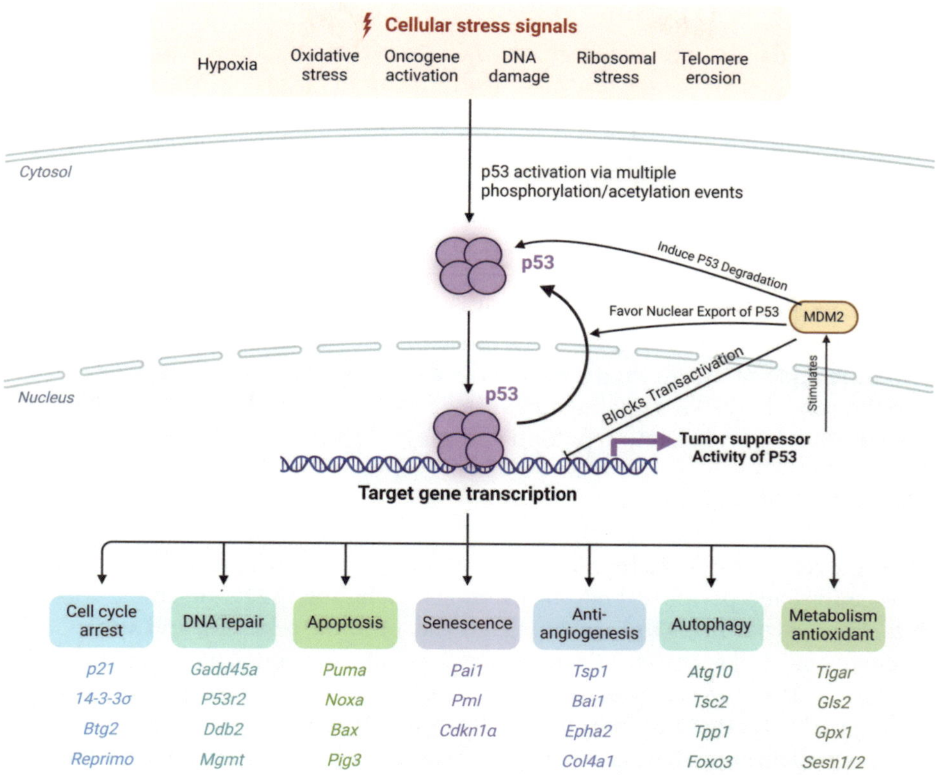

Figure 2.
The tumor suppressor protein p53 and its negative regulator MDM2 form an autoregulatory feedback loop that is critical for regulating p53 activity. p53 stimulates the expression of MDM2, while MDM2, in turn, inhibits p53 through multiple mechanisms including blocking its transcriptional functions, promoting its nuclear export, and targeting it for degradation. Cellular stress signals, such as DNA damage or oncogene activation, can disrupt the p53-MDM2 interaction and activate p53. For example, DNA damage induces phosphorylation of p53 that prevents it from binding MDM2, while oncogenic signals stimulate the ARF protein to inhibit MDM2-mediated p53 degradation. Small molecule inhibitors that block the interaction between p53 and MDM2 have been pursued as a strategy to reactivate wild type p53 function in tumor cells. However, these compounds could also potentially impact p53-independent functions of MDM2 that should be considered. Further, research is needed to fully elucidate the complex p53-MDM2 regulatory pathway and exploit it for therapeutic benefit in cancer.

destruction of insulin-producing beta cells occurs, necessitating exogenous insulin treatment. Type 2 diabetes involves peripheral insulin resistance coupled with inadequate compensatory insulin secretion, often associated with obesity. Several key signaling pathways governing glucose homeostasis and insulin action are impaired in diabetes. Binding of insulin to its receptor tyrosine kinase (RTK) leads to activation of cascades, such as PI3K/AKT and MAPK, that stimulate glucose uptake and storage. Insulin resistance in type 2 diabetes is linked to disruption of these pathways in skeletal muscle and adipose. The glucagon pathway activated by falling glucose levels signals the liver to increase glycogenolysis and gluconeogenesis *via* cAMP/PKA (protein kinase A—cAMP-dependent protein kinase that phosphorylates substrates involved in glycogen, sugar, and lipid metabolism) and other effectors. Dysregulation of this pathway contributes to uncontrolled glucose production in diabetes.

6.3 Cardiovascular disorders

Cardiovascular disorders are a group of diseases that affect the heart and blood vessels. These diseases are the leading cause of death in the world. Maladaptive signaling pathways that become chronically dysregulated in the cardiovascular system represent high-value targets for interrupting disease progression. The RAS/MAPK cascade activated by hypertension, inflammation, and stress can stimulate pathogenic vascular smooth muscle growth, leading to occlusive remodeling of arteries. Likewise, hyperactivation of pro-survival PI3K/AKT signals by insulin, glucose, and other metabolic stimuli may instigate the advancement of atherosclerotic cardiovascular disease. Furthermore, the inflammatory NF-κB pathway flared up by oxidative stress and immunological triggers can ignite damaging inflammatory responses in the vasculature and myocardium, provoking the development of heart disease.

Conversely, the PPAR signaling network governs beneficial lipid metabolism and homeostasis, with its activation potentializing cardioprotective effects (**Table 2**).

6.4 Neurological conditions

Neurological disorders encompass a broad range of debilitating conditions affecting the central and peripheral nervous systems, including the brain, spinal cord, and nerves. From Alzheimer's to Parkinson's disease, multiple sclerosis, and stroke, these heterogeneous diseases exact a tremendous physical, emotional, and economic toll on patients, families, and societies. Intensive research has uncovered several maladaptive signaling pathways that become chronically dysregulated in the damaged nervous system, representing potential targets for therapeutic interventions. For instance, in Alzheimer's disease, abnormal processing of amyloid precursor protein leads to

Pathway	Functions	Disease associations
RAS/MAPK	Cell growth, inflammation, fibrosis	Hypertension, cardiac hypertrophy
PI3K/AKT	Cell survival, metabolism, growth	Atherosclerosis, ischemia/reperfusion injury
eNOS/NO	Vascular relaxation, blood pressure regulation	Endothelial dysfunction
NF-κB	Inflammation	Atherosclerosis, diabetic complications
Wnt/β-catenin	Angiogenesis, cardiac remodeling	Heart failure
TGF-β/Smad	Fibrosis	Cardiac fibrosis, remodeling
Hippo	Cardiomyocyte proliferation, apoptosis, hypertrophy	Cardiac hypertrophy
cGMP/PKG	Vascular smooth muscle contraction	Impaired vasodilation
Cox-2/PGE2	Inflammation	Atherosclerotic plaque instability
JAK/STAT	Inflammation, angiogenesis, hypertension	Vascular inflammation, angiogenesis, hypertension

Table 2.
Table summarizing key signaling pathways involved in cardiovascular diseases.

Disease	Major signaling pathways involved
Alzheimer's disease	Amyloid cascade pathway (APP processing, amyloid-β accumulation) Tau phosphorylation pathway (tau aggregation, tangle formation) Neuroinflammation pathway (microglial activation, inflammatory mediators)
Parkinson's disease	Mitochondrial quality control pathways (PINK1/Parkin, mitophagy) Oxidative stress pathways (DJ-1, LRRK2, α-synuclein aggregation) Protein misfolding pathways (α-synuclein, Lewy body formation)
Multiple sclerosis	Myelin-associated glycoprotein pathway (complement activation) T cell pathway (T cell infiltration, autoimmunity) B cell pathway (antibody production against myelin)
Amyotrophic lateral sclerosis	Oxidative stress pathways Glutamate excitotoxicity pathways Protein aggregation pathways Axonal transport pathways RNA metabolism pathways
Huntington's disease	Synaptic signaling dysfunction (BDNF, dopamine) Transcriptional dysregulation Mitochondrial dysfunction Excitotoxicity (NMDA receptor)
Stroke	Inflammation pathways (TNF-α, IL-1β, IL-6) Apoptosis pathways (p53, Bcl2, caspases) Oxidative stress pathways Blood-brain barrier dysfunction pathways
Epilepsy	Ion channel mutations (Na^+, K^+, Ca^{2+}, Cl^- channels) mTOR pathway Neuroinflammation pathways GABAergic signaling deficits

Table 3.
Signaling pathways involvement in neurological conditions.

accumulation of neurotoxic amyloid beta plaques *via* the amyloid cascade pathway. This pathway triggers downstream neuroinflammation and cell death signaling. Likewise, aberrant hyperphosphorylation of the microtubule-associated protein tau activates pathways causing it to misfold and aggregate within neurons, also eliciting destructive inflammation.

Furthermore, chronic activation of microglia, the resident immune cells in the central nervous system, provokes runway neuroinflammatory signaling contributing to neurodegeneration. Mitochondrial damage can also ignite vicious cycles of reactive oxygen species production and energetic crisis in nerve cells. Conversely, deficient trophic signaling due to lowered neurotrophic factors compromises neuronal health and survival (**Table 3**).

7. Biosignaling and targeted therapy

As knowledge of signaling pathways expands, targeted therapies promise to transform treatment paradigms by addressing root causes of disease, rather than just suppressing symptoms. Matching targeted drugs to the molecular profiles of patients also sets the stage for a new era of personalized medicine.

7.1 Approaches to targeting signaling pathways

See **Table 4**.

It is important to note that there is no single approach to targeting signaling pathways that is best for all diseases. The best approach will depend on the specific disease and the signaling pathway that is involved.

Approach	Description	Examples
Small molecule inhibitors	Small molecules that inhibit specific components of signaling pathways.	Tyrosine kinase inhibitors (e.g., Imatinib for BCR-ABL in chronic myeloid leukemia)
		BRAF inhibitors (e.g., Vemurafenib for BRAF-mutant melanoma)
Monoclonal antibodies	Antibodies designed to target specific receptors or ligands involved in signaling pathways.	Trastuzumab (Herceptin) targeting HER2 in breast cancer. Rituximab targeting CD20 in B-cell lymphomas other examples are rituximab and infliximab.
Gene therapy	The delivery of therapeutic genes to modify or correct signaling pathway components.	Adeno-associated virus (AAV) vectors deliver normal genes to treat genetic diseases. CRISPR-Cas technology for gene editing to correct mutations. Other examples: Glybera, Kymriah, and Luxturna.
RNA interference (RNAi)	Silencing specific genes using RNA molecules to disrupt signaling pathway components.	siRNA targeting oncogenes in cancer therapy and inhibit TTR synthesis in polyneuropathy. Examples: Patisiran, givosiran.
Immune checkpoint inhibitors	Blockade of immune checkpoint proteins to enhance immune response against tumors.	Pembrolizumab and nivolumab targeting PD-1 in cancer immunotherapy. Ipilimumab targeting CTLA-4 in melanoma treatment.
Nanoparticle delivery	Utilizing nanoparticles to deliver targeted therapies to specific cells or tissues.	Liposomal doxorubicin for cancer-targeted drug delivery. Dendrimers delivering drugs across the blood-brain barrier.
Small molecule inhibitors	Chemically synthesized compounds that permeate cells and bind to specific intracellular proteins, such as kinases to inhibit signaling.	Imatinib, gefitinib, vemurafenib
Antisense oligonucleotides	Bind to RNA sequences to alter gene expression and signaling protein levels.	Nusinersen, eteplirsen

Table 4.
Table of various approaches targeting signaling pathways.

8. Investigating cell signaling pathways

Cell signaling pathways comprise intricate molecular circuits that govern critical cellular processes such as growth, differentiation, and survival. Abnormalities in signaling underlie many diseases. A range of techniques exist to study signaling cascades, which can be broadly classified as *in silico* computational approaches or *in vitro* experimental approaches.

8.1 *In vitro* techniques

In vitro, biochemical and cell-based assays directly analyze signaling proteins and responses. Immunoblotting tracks protein activation states. Reporter gene assays couple signaling responses to measurable outputs. Fluorescence microscopy visualizes protein localization. Flow cytometry quantifies signaling-induced changes in cellular states. Chromatin immunoprecipitation detects DNA binding of activated transcription factors. Genetic manipulation with CRISPR screens perturbs signaling nodes. Miniaturized lab-on-a-chip devices enable high-throughput analysis. Together, these experimental tools provide multifaceted insight into pathway mechanics.

8.1.1 Molecular assays

Molecular assays allow direct measurement of the levels and activities of signaling components such as mRNAs, proteins, and metabolites. By quantifying pathway participants, molecular assays elucidate signaling mechanisms and identify dysregulated nodes.

8.1.1.1 Western blotting

Detects specific proteins within cell lysates using antibodies. Shows protein expression levels and modifications, such as phosphorylation critical for pathway activation. Quantitative blotting enables comparison of signaling protein activation states between samples.

8.1.1.2 Co-immunoprecipitation

Utilizes antibody-based purification of protein complexes to identify signaling protein interactions and binding partners through mass spectrometry. Reveals pathway connectivity and multiprotein signaling nodes.

8.1.1.3 Enzyme-linked immunosorbent assay (ELISA)

Quantifies protein targets using antibodies coupled to colorimetric or fluorescent readouts. Enables high-throughput measurement of circulating intracellular signaling proteins secreted into bodily fluids as potential biomarkers of pathway activation.

8.1.1.4 qPCR

Measures gene expression levels through sequence-specific fluorescent probes. Identifies transcriptional targets induced by activated signaling cascades. Highly sensitive for detecting subtle pathway effects on gene networks.

8.1.1.5 RNA sequencing

Provides comprehensive transcriptomic profiles, showing global effects of signaling on gene expression. Bioinformatic analysis elucidates coordinated differential gene expression patterns induced by pathways.

Molecular assays provide multifaceted, often highly sensitive means to directly analyze abundance and activities of signaling components. Integration of results from orthogonal assays gives comprehensive and quantitative insight into intricate pathway dynamics.

8.2 *In silico* techniques

In silico, techniques utilize computational methods to analyze high-throughput omics datasets and map signaling networks. Gene expression profiling, proteomics, and RNAi screening can identify components and connectivity within pathways. Network modeling based on protein-protein interactions predicts signaling topology and dynamic behaviors. Pathway enrichment analysis discovers coordinated gene sets. Machine learning classifies cell states based on signaling patterns. These computational tools enable rapid analysis of complex pathways.

8.2.1 Proteomics

Proteomics is a discipline focused on the comprehensive identification and quantification of all proteins expressed within a biological system. This approach goes beyond mere enumeration, delving into the structural intricacies, functional interactions, and cellular locations of proteins in physiological and pathological contexts [18]. Utilizing advanced techniques, such as high-resolution mass spectrometry and multidimensional liquid chromatography, proteomics provides detailed insights into signaling networks [19]. It reveals the dynamics, feedback mechanisms, and intersections of signaling molecules, offering valuable information about potential therapeutic targets, dysregulations, and redundancies [20]. In the field of drug discovery and translational medicine, proteomics plays a crucial role by uncovering unknown protein targets, deciphering protein-drug interactions, and highlighting unintended off-target effects of therapeutic agents [21].

8.3 Pathway analysis tools

Pathway analysis tools are bioinformatics resources that identify, map, and analyze the complex molecular networks that comprise signaling cascades. These tools integrate multidimensional omics data to elucidate pathway components, connectivity, dynamics, and disease associations.

a. *BioCarta* is a web-based platform with over 300 curated signaling maps, derived from literature reviews, highlighting gene and protein interactions and their associations with diseases [22, 23].

b. *KEGG* is a commercial pathway database that maps pathways for various organisms based on literature curation, linking them to sequence, chemical, and disease data [24].

c. *Reactome* is an open-access pathway knowledgebase focused on human pathways, incorporating detailed molecular maps with protein interactions, subcellular locations, and posttranslational modifications [25].

d. *Ingenuity pathway analysis* is a commonly used commercial tool that analyzes user omics data in the context of an expert-curated database, identifying enriched pathways and upstream regulators [26]. It generates interactive networks and requires a site license purchase but offers a free trial access option.

9. Challenges and limitations

Challenges in developing drugs targeting signaling pathways, including drug resistance and off-target effects:

9.1 Drug resistance

A major obstacle limiting targeted therapies is the eventual emergence of drug resistance, whereby tumors become insensitive to the drug through a variety of mechanisms [27]. Alterations in the drug binding site through mutations prevent drug interaction with the target. Activation of compensatory signaling pathways circumvents the inhibited cascade. Efflux pumps eject the drug from cancer cells. Combination therapies blocking multiple nodes in a pathway or parallel pathways can delay resistance by eliminating escape routes. New drugs are also being designed to inhibit mutated target variants [28]. Understanding and targeting the specific genomic and phenotypic changes enabling resistance holds promise for overcoming this challenge.

9.2 Off-target effects

The promise of targeted therapies lies in their selective modulation of pathways driving disease. However, unintended binding at off-target sites results in side effects and safety liabilities, posing a second key challenge. Highly specific drugs minimize interactions at off-target proteins. Screening chemical libraries early in development weeds out promiscuous compounds. Prodrugs activated locally release drugs predominantly at tumor sites [29]. Nanoparticles accumulate preferentially in tumors, sparing normal tissues. Comprehensive toxicity evaluation in preclinical models defines risks and guides treatment planning. Overall, designing exquisitely selective targeted drugs, minimizing systemic exposure, and rigorous safety testing help reduce the potential for adverse off-target effects [30].

10. Future directions

In future directions of signaling pathway research, several key areas hold promise for advancing drug development. Integration of omics data, including genomics, transcriptomics, proteomics, and metabolomics, can provide a more detailed understanding of signaling networks and aid in the identification of therapeutic targets. Systems biology approaches, such as mathematical modeling and computational simulations, offer valuable tools for predicting pathway behavior and optimizing drug interventions. Single-cell analysis techniques allow for the study of cellular heterogeneity, enabling the development of targeted therapies that address diverse signaling profiles. Furthermore, exploring noncanonical signaling pathways and investigating combination therapies that target multiple pathways simultaneously show potential for overcoming drug resistance and improving treatment outcomes. Bridging the gap between basic research and clinical practice through translational research efforts will aid in the development of biomarkers and clinical trials for targeted therapies. These future directions have the potential to revolutionize drug development and lead to more effective therapeutic interventions.

11. Conclusion

The emerging opportunities for targeting signaling pathways represent a new frontier brimming with possibilities for transforming drug development and advancing precision medicine. As researchers, we stand at an inflection point where revolutionary technologies can be combined with comprehensive molecular insights to open new therapeutic avenues. Gene editing tools may 1 day provide curative solutions by correcting pathological mutations in signaling cascades. The burgeoning field of immuno-oncology demonstrates how we can harness the body's own defenses to target aberrant pathways driving cancer. Nanomedicines offer targeted delivery capabilities to increase the precision of signaling modulation, and artificial intelligence empowers rapid in silico drug design and predictive informatics. Equally important is embracing personalized medicine approaches, where therapies are matched to the specific signaling disruptions in each patient. Integrating large-scale profiling, computational analysis, and functional screening will enable patient-tailored targeting of pathways. To fully realize this vision, we must foster strong interdisciplinary collaboration across fields and industry-academia partnerships to accelerate translation. Expanding funding for signaling research and adapting regulatory policies will also be critical to support these emerging opportunities. The future is bright as we are poised to unlock the full potential of signaling pathways for drug discovery. But there is much work ahead. As researchers, we must drive forward innovations in this space to usher in a new era of precision medicine, where targeted therapies shaped by a deep understanding of signaling circuits can deliver improved outcomes for patients. The possibilities make this an incredibly exciting time to be exploring new frontiers in targeting signaling pathways.

Author details

Habab Ali Ahmad, Kiran Seemab, Fazal Wahab and Muhammad Imran Khan*
Pak-Austria Fachhochschule Institute of Applied Sciences and Technology, Haripur, Khyber Pakhtunkhwa, Pakistan

*Address all correspondence to: mik8782@gmail.com

References

[1] El-Mahdy HA et al. miRNAs role in bladder cancer pathogenesis and targeted therapy: Signaling pathways interplay—A review. Pathology, Research and Practice. 2023;**242**:154316

[2] Levonen A-L et al. Antioxidant gene therapy for cardiovascular disease: Current status and future perspectives. Circulation. 2008;**117**(16):2142-2150

[3] Liu Q et al. Small molecules from natural sources, targeting signaling pathways in diabetes. Biochimica et Biophysica Acta (BBA)-Gene Regulatory Mechanisms. 2010;**1799**(10-12):854-865

[4] Ahluwalia K et al. Lipidomics in understanding pathophysiology and pharmacologic effects in inflammatory diseases: Considerations for drug development. Metabolites. 2022;**12**(4):333

[5] Nojeem L et al. Uncovering the complexity of cell signaling pathways using systems biology approaches. American-Eurasian Journal of Scientific Research. 2023;**2023**(**11**):131-135

[6] Bertucci A, Bertucci F, Gonçalves A. Phosphoinositide 3-kinase (PI3K) inhibitors and breast cancer: An overview of current achievements. Cancers. 2023;**15**(5):1416

[7] Gazdar AF. Personalized medicine and inhibition of EGFR signaling in lung cancer. The New England Journal of Medicine. 2009;**361**(10):1018

[8] Wang N et al. Emerging role of ERBB2 in targeted therapy for metastatic colorectal cancer: Signaling pathways to therapeutic strategies. Cancers. 2022;**14**(20):5160

[9] Pan Q et al. Recent advances in boosting EGFR tyrosine kinase inhibitors-based cancer therapy. Molecular Pharmaceutics. 2023;**20**(2):829-852

[10] Zhang M et al. Targeted therapy for autoimmune diseases based on multifunctional frame nucleic acid system: Blocking TNF-α-NF-κB signaling and mediating macrophage polarization. Chemical Engineering Journal. 2023;**454**:140399

[11] Ding Q et al. Signaling pathways in rheumatoid arthritis: Implications for targeted therapy. Signal Transduction and Targeted Therapy. 2023;**8**(1):68

[12] Kumar V, Bauer C, Stewart JH IV. Cancer cell-specific cGAS/STING signaling pathway in the era of advancing cancer cell biology. European Journal of Cell Biology. 2023;**102**(3):151338

[13] Al-Qudah MA et al. Correlation of PKM2 expression with HER2/neu and additional breast cancer biomarkers and its prognostic significance. Applied Immunohistochemistry & Molecular Morphology. 2023;**31**(6):363-370

[14] Lopetuso LR et al. Focus on anti-tumour necrosis factor (TNF)-α-related autoimmune diseases. International Journal of Molecular Sciences. 2023;**24**(9):8187

[15] Li J et al. PHPB attenuated cognitive impairment in type 2 diabetic KK-Ay mice by modulating SIRT1/insulin signaling pathway and inhibiting generation of AGEs. Pharmaceuticals. 2023;**16**(2):305

[16] Journo C et al. NRP/optineurin cooperates with TAX1BP1 to potentiate

the activation of NF-κB by human T-lymphotropic virus type 1 tax protein. PLoS Pathogens. 2009;**5**(7):e1000521

[17] Piccolo S, Dupont S, Cordenonsi M. The biology of YAP/TAZ: Hippo signaling and beyond. Physiological Reviews. 2014;**94**(4):1287-1312

[18] Mann M, Jensen ON. Proteomic analysis of post-translational modifications. Nature Biotechnology. 2003;**21**(3):255-261

[19] Cox J, Mann M. Quantitative, high-resolution proteomics for data-driven systems biology. Annual Review of Biochemistry. 2011;**80**:273-299

[20] Zhang Y et al. Protein analysis by shotgun/bottom-up proteomics. Chemical Reviews. 2013;**113**(4):2343-2394

[21] Han G et al. Large-scale phosphoproteome analysis of human liver tissue by enrichment and fractionation of phosphopeptides with strong anion exchange chromatography. Proteomics. 2008;**8**(7):1346-1361

[22] Turenne N. Role of a web-based software platform for systems biology. Journal of Computer Science and Systems Biology. 2011;**4**:035-041

[23] Nishimura D. BioCarta. Biotech Software & Internet Report: The Computer Software Journal for Scientists. 2001;**2**(3):117-120

[24] Kanehisa M. The KEGG database. In: 'In silico' Simulation of Biological Processes: Novartis Foundation Symposium. Vol. 247. Chichester, UK: John Wiley & Sons, Ltd.; 15 Nov 2002. pp. 91-103

[25] Fabregat A et al. The reactome pathway knowledgebase. Nucleic Acids Research. 2018;**46**(D1):D649-D655

[26] Krämer A et al. Causal analysis approaches in ingenuity pathway analysis. Bioinformatics. 2014;**30**(4):523-530

[27] Holohan C et al. Cancer drug resistance: An evolving paradigm. Nature Reviews Cancer. 2013;**13**(10):714-726

[28] Poornima P et al. Network pharmacology of cancer: From understanding of complex interactomes to the design of multi-target specific therapeutics from nature. Pharmacological Research. 2016;**111**:290-302

[29] Davis MI et al. Comprehensive analysis of kinase inhibitor selectivity. Nature Biotechnology. 2011;**29**(11):1046-1051

[30] Cavagnaro JA. Preclinical safety evaluation of biotechnology-derived pharmaceuticals. Nature Reviews Drug Discovery. 2002;**1**(6):469-475

Chapter 5

Neuroprotection Mediated by Prolactin during Excitotoxicity: New Functions and Insights

Gladys Molina-Salinas, Valeria Rodríguez-Chávez and Marco Cerbón

Abstract

Prolactin (PRL) is a peptide and pleiotropic hormone with more than 300 associated functions such as maternal behavior, lactation, osmoregulation, angiogenesis, and the immune system. It is associated with several functions in the brain, including lactation, cognition and memory, maternal behavior, and neurogenesis. PRL reportedly plays an important role in neuroprotection against excitotoxicity caused by glutamate (Glu) and kainic acid (KA) damage *in vitro* and *in vivo* models. However, the molecular mechanisms involved in the neuroprotective effects of PRL are unclear. Despite this, data suggest the involvement of PI3K/AKT, and GSK3β/NF-κB signaling pathways, which are involved in neuroprotection. In addition, PRL inhibits Glu- and KA-induced increase by intracellular Ca^{2+} concentration, leading to neuronal survival. We also discuss current knowledge on the role of PRL in neurodegenerative diseases. New avenues of research into the protective mechanisms of PRL and its potential therapeutic effects on the brain under pathological and physiological conditions are needed.

Keywords: prolactin, neuroprotection, excitotoxicity, signaling pathways, calcium regulation, NMDA/AMPA channels, neurogenerative disease

1. Introduction

Current research aims to find molecules or compounds that are capable of protecting cells from damage and subsequent cell death, which may cause pathophysiology or neurodegenerative diseases (NDs) [1–4]. Excitotoxicity is cell damage that can trigger death by apoptosis and necrosis and is involved in multiple neurological conditions, including epilepsy, stroke, and neurodegenerative disorders [4–7]. These neurological conditions are a heterogeneous group of diseases with different clinical phenotypes and genetic etiologies that are characterized by the gradual loss of specific populations of neuronal cells and dysfunction of proteins that influence several signaling cascades that cause neuronal damage [1, 4–6]. In addition, these conditions share common pathogenic mechanisms, including the deregulation of intracellular calcium (Ca^{2+})

homeostasis, the activation of nitric oxide synthesis, and the activation of reactive oxygen species (ROS), which damage different biomolecules (lipids, proteins, carbohydrates, and nucleic acids), altering cell function and inducing cell death, leading to progressive neurodegeneration [1, 8, 9]. However, there are few natural compounds capable of exerting neuroprotective effects against excitotoxicity such as curcumin [10], vitamins [11], and hormones. Recently, prolactin (PRL), a peptide hormone, has been in the limelight for its role in neuroprotective processes [1, 12–14]. PRL is relevant due to its neuroprotective effects *in vivo* and *in vitro* models; however, its mechanism of action has not been completely described [1, 13–16]. Therefore, the aim of this chapter is to understand the role of PRL-induced neuroprotection in NDs and to highlight the latest knowledge on the role of PRL in NDs and neuroprotective mechanisms.

2. Prolactin

To understand the neuroprotective effects of PRL, it is necessary to know its characteristics and mechanism of action. Since its discovery in the 1930s by the biologist Oscar Riddle [17, 18], it has been considered a hormone that controls the production and secretion of milk, and nowadays, it is known as a multifunctional endocrine hormone of great interest in the scientific community [19, 20].

PRL is known to have strong structural homology with growth hormone and placental lactogen, which belongs to a large family of hematopoietic cytokine proteins characterized by having a tertiary structure composed of four antiparallel α-helices [21, 22]. Likewise, the mature PRL protein of pituitary origin is composed of 197 and 199 amino acids in rats and humans, respectively, with three disulfide bonds located in similar positions in both species [19, 23]. It is widely accepted that PRL is synthesized in the anterior lobe of the pituitary by specialized cells called lactotrophs [21, 24, 25]. It is now known that it can also be produced by other extrapituitary cells [16, 26, 27]. In addition, transcriptional regulation of pituitary and extrapituitary PRL expressions are controlled by a proximal and a distal promoter region, respectively [16, 22, 27].

PRL is present in all mammals [22, 23, 28] and is encoded by a single gene (PRL) composed of five exons and four introns in the majority of the species [22, 25]. Nevertheless, at the molecular level, its expression and regulation are tissue-specific because several isoforms have been described that result from proteolytic cleavages, alternative splicing, or posttranslational modifications, such as glycosylation, phosphorylation, deamidation, and association with other circulating proteins, thus modifying its biological activity [16, 21, 29].

PRL can have various forms of modification, for example, high molecular mass PRL, such as "big PRL" and "big big PRL" (also known as macroprolactin) of approximately 100 kDa; however, these forms show lower activity and could participate in the storage, modification, and release of PRL [16, 21]. There are those with low molecular mass of 14, 16, and 22 kDa that are generated from proteolytic cleavage of the 23 kDa pituitary PRL [17, 18, 22]. In addition, PRL can form dimers, polymers, and aggregates, and its actions are mediated by its receptor [18, 29]. See **Figure 1** where the PRL structure and its receptor are described.

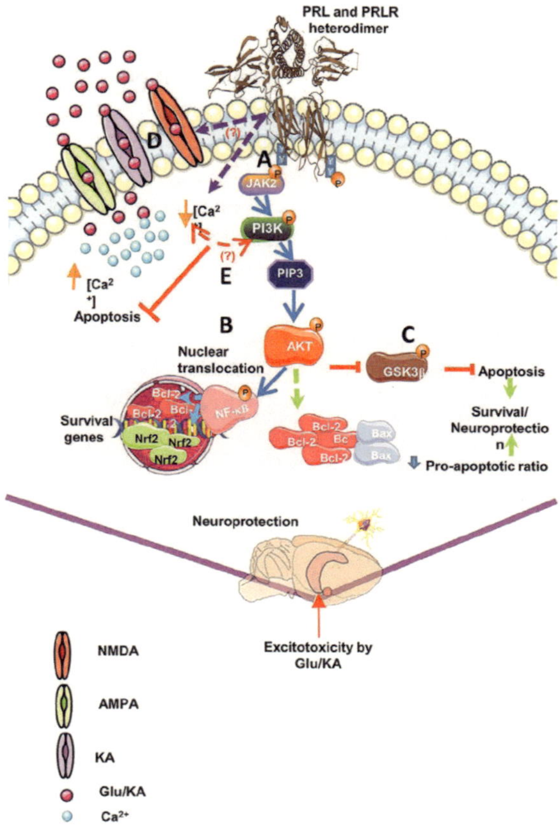

Figure 1.
The possible molecular mechanisms of action of PRL-induced neuroprotection against excitotoxic damage. (A) the PRLR heterodimer binds to its ligand activating the JAK2 kinase, which phosphorylates PI3K, subsequently it promotes the activation of AKT. The blue line shows the activation of PI3K/AKT signaling pathway (B) which may promote NF-κB translocation to the nucleus increasing expression of survival genes, such as Nrf2 and Bcl-2, it promotes a reduction in the proapoptotic ratio. (C) AKT inhibits GSK3β, which is involved in apoptotic events. (D) NMDA, Glu and KA channels allow massive calcium influx in response to excitotoxicity events induced by excess Glu or KA, that increases intracellular calcium concentration, leading to neuronal damage such as apoptosis. (E) PRL could bind to NMDA, Glu and KA receptors to inhibit excitotoxicity-induced by a massive intracellular calcium entry. Consequently, it could mitigate apoptosis, then this down-regulation of intracellular calcium by PRL could be related to its interaction with signaling pathways (?). AKT: protein kinase B; Bcl-2: B-cell lymphoma 2; Glu: glutamate; GSK3β: glycogen synthase kinase-3; JAK2: Janus kinase-2; KA: kainic acid; NMDA: N-methyl-D-aspartate receptor; NF-κB: factor κ-light-chain-enhancer of activated B cells; PI3K: phosphatidylinositol 3-kinase; PIP3: phosphatidylinositol (3,4,5)-triphosphate; PRL: prolactin; and PRLR: prolactin receptor. Modified from Molina-Salinas et al. [30].

3. Prolactin receptors

PRL actions are initiated by binding to a homodimer of the prolactin receptor (PRLR), forming a heterotrimeric complex with the ligand [27, 29].

Rat and human PRLRs are membrane proteins belonging to the class I cytokine receptor superfamily [16, 27, 29]. These receptors are single-pass transmembrane proteins that lack intrinsic tyrosine kinase activity and can be phosphorylated by cytoplasmic proteins

[16, 27, 29]. They are composed of three domains: extracellular, with two regions, designated S1 and S2 (or D1 and D2) that together form the ligand binding site; transmembrane, which is identical in both species; and intracellular or cytoplasmic, of variable length and composition [20, 22, 27, 28]. PRLRs are mainly related to the activation of the JAK2-STAT5 signaling pathway but can initiate other signaling cascades, in addition to being ubiquitously expressed in various tissues [16, 24, 29].

Multiple PRLR isoforms resulting from alternative splicing of the primary mRNA transcript have been identified in rodents and humans [22, 29, 31]. These isoforms have identical extracellular and transmembrane domains, only differing in length and sequence in the intracellular domains [20, 32]. Three different isoforms of PRLRs have been identified in rats: short (PRLR-S), intermediate (PRLR-I), and long (PRLR-L) [16, 22], while a soluble isoform has been described in humans. The most studied isoforms are the PRLR-L, PRLR-I, and PRLR-S due to their distribution and expression [16, 27].

Regarding the PRL activation pathway, the binding of PRL to the PRLR-L triggers different signaling pathways, the main signaling cascade being *via* the (JAK2/STAT5) pathway [22, 27, 31]. It should be noted that the discovery of this pathway was a great advance in the understanding of PRL actions [22, 33, 34]. PRL can also induce the activation of at least two other pathways, MAPK/ERK1/2 and P13K/AKT, and the activation of all these pathways can influence the previously described functions of PRL [16, 25, 35].

Finally, it should be noted that the PRLR is expressed in several tissues such as the mammary gland, gonads, liver, kidneys, adrenal gland, brain, heart, lungs, pituitary gland, uterus, skeletal muscle, skin, and cells of the immune system [16, 18, 23, 25, 29]. Despite being found in many tissues, this article focuses on PRLR expression in the brain, where it has been reported in several brain areas such as the olfactory bulb, corpus callosum, choroid plexuses, amygdala, hypothalamus, thalamus, cerebral cortex, and hippocampus [15, 27, 29].

4. Prolactin functions

Although PRL has been predominantly related to pituitary lactotrophs, it is now recognized that it is also expressed and secreted in other tissues [22, 23, 25]. Therefore, it is considered a pleiotropic hormone with more than 300 known physiological effects [22, 23] such as reproduction, lactogenesis, immunomodulation, angiogenesis, energy metabolism, osmotic balance, and development regulation [27, 35, 36]. It has also been reported that PRL can cross the blood-brain barrier [26, 36], and its effects on the brain depend on factors such as age, sex, and reproductive status of the species [27, 31]. Importantly, PRL has been reported to regulate specific neuronal circuits and participate in many brain functions, including maternal behavior, energy balance, food intake, sleep, anxiety, neurogenesis, migraine, and pain [16, 18, 36–38].

Interestingly, a transcriptomic analysis by Cabrera-Reyes et al. [15] indicated that PRL induces the expression of different sets of genes involved in brain processes related to learning, behavior, memory, neuroprotection, neurodevelopment, neurogenesis, remodeling, plasticity, and sleep/wake-up regulation.

5. Prolactin in neuroprotection

As mentioned above, PRL is related to more than 300 biological actions, highlighting its role as a neuroprotective hormone against excitotoxicity, which has been described in both *in vivo* and *in vitro* models [1, 12–15, 39].

The concept of excitotoxicity was originally suggested by Olney et al. [40] to refer to the ability of glutamate (Glu) to induce neuronal damage [41]. Nowadays, this term generally refers to neuronal injury and death, resulting from prolonged exposure to Glu and excitatory amino acids [2, 42]. This exposure induces overactivation of ionotropic glutamatergic neuronal receptors such as α-amino-3-hydroxy-5-methyl-4-isoxazolepropionic acid receptor, N-methyl-D-aspartate receptor, and kainic acid [43, 44]. Overactivation causes an increase in Ca^{2+} intracellular concentration, which, in turn, induces the activation of Ca^{2+}-dependent enzymes and the generation of free radicals (ROS). When there is an excessive increase in Ca^{2+} and ROS, mitochondrial membrane potential decreases, releasing mitochondrial factors Cytochrome-C and apoptosis-inducing factor, triggering apoptosome complex activation *via* caspases, which leads to nuclear condensation and DNA fragmentation [8, 9, 15, 45, 46] Glu and KA are capable of inducing cell death by apoptosis and necrosis *in vivo* and *in vitro* models [12, 47].

Cabrera-Reyes et al. [15] used *in vivo* models to show that PRL significantly modifies microglial morphology, reduces Cd11b/c protein expression, and alters the content and location of the neuronal proteins Tau, Map2, and Syp, which intervene in axogenic and synaptic functions. It has also been reported that PRL can act as an endogenous anxiolytic agent, capable of inducing dose-dependent suppression of anxiety behaviors, as well as acute stress response [23, 36, 48].

Beside, neuroprotection by PRL was analyzed using primary cultures of hippocampal neurons, proving that the hormone performs its functions through interaction with its receptor [13] and that administrating PRL before excitotoxic damage by Glu prevents cell death and mitochondrial dysfunction, inhibits the increase in intracellular Ca^{2+} levels triggered by the excitotoxic insult, and promotes the activation of the transcriptional factor NF-κB, which induces overexpression of the antiapoptotic protein Bcl-2 in hippocampal neurons [14]. In addition, molecular signaling pathways, involving PI3K/AKT and NF-κB/GSK3β, could be implicated in the molecular mechanisms that explain the effects of PRL against excitotoxicity and neuroprotection [14, 16, 27].

Recently, Molina-Salinas et al. [30] demonstrated that PRL activates the PI3K/AKT signaling pathway during Glu excitotoxicity, which promotes neuronal survival through AKT activation and GSK3β/NF-κB upregulation, resulting in the induction of *Bcl-2* and *Nrf2* gene expression. In addition, inhibition of the PI3K/AKT signaling pathway abrogated the protective effect of PRL against Glu-induced neuronal death. Furthermore, another study found that administering PRL induced a significant increase in neuronal viability after KA treatment and decreased intracellular Ca^{2+} concentrations induced by KA treatment, suggesting that PRL can generate a neuroprotective effect by modifying Ca^{2+} cell homeostasis [49]. **Figure 1** shows possible molecular mechanisms of prolactin to induce neuroprotection against excitotoxicity. It is important to note that although PRL can act as a neuroprotective agent [21, 22, 29, 35]. These effects will be discussed later in this chapter.

6. Prolactin and its relation to neurodegenerative diseases

NDs have a common characteristic; the progressive loss of neuronal populations due to the changes in their structure and function [50] that lead to neuronal death. These pathologies also have similar cellular mechanisms and histopathological features [51] identified as an aberrant protein process and in their trafficking and aggregation in neurons by dysregulation in their ubiquitin–proteasomal and autophagosome/lysosomal systems. Other mechanisms include the formation of extracellular plaques that induce neuroinflammation through microglia activation [52–54] and increase oxidative stress levels that result in neuronal progressive damage. Moreover, as discussed previously, excitotoxicity is involved in NDs [42, 55].

NDs may be grouped based on their similarities: first, clinical features related to the anatomic distribution of neurodegeneration (frontotemporal degenerations, extrapyramidal disorders, or spinocerebellar degenerations), and second, by protein biochemical abnormalities [56, 57]. It is well-known that the most common NDs are amyloidosis, tauopathies, and α-synucleinopathies [58]. Interestingly, these protein abnormalities can be present before clinical manifestations begin. Therefore, it is important to find new treatments and develop strategies against these diseases. In this sense, PRL as a neuroprotective agent may play a role against neurodegenerative pathologies. In the next sections, we will discuss how PRL participates in these diseases.

6.1 Evidence of the role of prolactin in Alzheimer's disease

Alzheimer's disease (AD) is a well-known chronic neurodegenerative disease whose main targeted brain areas are the medial temporal lobe and associative neocortical structures. Over the years hallmarks of AD, research have been described, among them is the accumulation of the amyloid-beta peptide (Aβ) in the brain, which results in aggregation of this insoluble oligomer and protofibrils. Moreover, cytoskeletal changes derived from hyperphosphorylation of microtubule-associated Tau protein in neurons are a feature. Overproduction of Aβ results from a failure in proteolytic cleavage of the amyloid precursor protein (APP). Accumulation of fibrillary Aβ results in senility and neurotic plaque formation. This event and the incapability of Aβ clearance from the brain trigger an extracellular accumulation of Aβ, and consequently oxidative stress, cytoskeletal changes, neuronal dysfunction, and finally neuronal death [59–61].

In a pioneering study describing PRL regulation in AD patients with dementia, subjects referred to as having Alzheimer's senile dementia (SDAT) and their respective control were treated with metoclopramide (a dopamine-blocking drug). The results showed no difference in PRL levels between patients with dementia and controls after 24 hours of treatment. However, 30 min after metoclopramide injection, PRL levels increased significantly, suggesting that PRL regulation in dementia caused by AD is controlled through the tuberoinfundibular pathway [62].

In contrast, successive studies have reported that serum PRL levels do not respond to thyrotropin-releasing hormone (TRH) stimulation in subjects with multi-infarct dementia and patients with SDAT. Indeed, PRL concentration was similar in these types of dementia. In addition, the authors reported that there was no correlation between dementia degradation and PRL level [63]. Despite the limitations of these studies due to the small number of patients included, an interesting relationship between dementia caused by AD and serum/plasma PRL concentrations was found. However, the correlation between PRL and AD has not yet been studied in depth, and other risk factors, such as age and sex, have not been considered in these investigations.

Other evidence supporting PRL participation in the pathophysiology of neurological diseases was reported in a common AD model with APPswe/PS1dE9 double transgenic male murine. PRL and PRLR genes were downregulated during the early stages of amyloidogenesis in the hippocampus compared to wild-type mice [64], suggesting that PRL possibly participates in the pathophysiology of AD.

In this regard, PRL has been associated with regulating some proteins and even signaling pathways that may be involved in the development and progression of AD, such as the case of glycogen synthase kinase-3 (GSK3). In AD, the PI3K/AKT signaling pathway is reduced, its inactivity leads to increased hyperphosphorylation of Tau, which is important for microtubule stability [65, 66]. AKT promotes GSK3 inhibition and subsequent reduction of Tau phosphorylation. Inactivation of GSK3 correlates with elevated levels of PRLR protein [67], which could explain in part why a lower concentration of PRL is associated with AD. Notably, AKT is one of the main signaling pathways used by PRL in the brain [16].

In addition, PRL displays a neuroprotective role mediated by Tau regulation during female neurodegeneration in response to PI3K/AKT/GSK3β pathway activation [68] and may promote neuronal survival [30]. Moreover, lactation as a physiological process induces a regulation of GSK3-α and p-Tau levels in lactating rats exposed to restraint stress. Lactating rats that were sacrificed 24 h after exposure to restraint stress had an increase of p-Tau in contrast to the restraint-stressed lactating rats sacrificed only 20 min after stress exposure, which showed reduced phosphorylation levels [69]. Thus, these experiments suggest that the regulatory dynamics between PRL hormone and GSK3 expression might play a role in AD pathology.

Another association between PRL and NDs is TRH, which is a well-known regulator of PRL secretion in tuberoinfundibular dopamine neurons [70, 71]. Like other hormones, such as PRL, TRH administration has been studied in neuroprotection [72]. It has been reported that reduction of GSK3β activity induced a reduction of Tau phosphorylation, and TRH gene depletion promoted the highest levels of GSK3β protein in cultured rat hippocampal neurons. Interestingly, the downregulation of TRH and its receptors has been implicated as a risk factor for developing AD and dementia [73–75]. Moreover, in women, the lowest and highest levels of serum TSH concentrations increased the risk of developing AD, but this correlation was not observed in men [76]. These observations suggest the possible sex-differential role that hormones play in neurodegenerative conditions.

Diverse approaches to identifying possible biomarkers as therapy triggers for AD have been reported [77]. Interestingly, PRL was proposed as a biomarker in a novel study showing a robust protein analyte from data of three cohorts to find analytes using Aβ1–42 in cerebrospinal fluid (CSF). PRL level was higher in patients with low Aβ1–42 levels compared to other groups [78]. Although this study suggests a possible involvement of PRL in AD pathology, the authors propose further studies to determine its usefulness in diagnosis and benefits in the treatment of AD.

On the other hand, melatonin, cortisol, homocysteine, and PRL plasma concentrations were measured in 85 patients. Notably, increased levels of PRL plasma were reported in subjects with AD and dementia [79]. Beside, a study indicated that both women and men with AD showed an increase in TSH, PRL, and GH plasma levels [60]. Conversely, in another study with elderly patients over 60 years, PRL serum levels did not change significantly [80]. These studies highlight the difficulty of using

PRL diagnosis or even to determine the progression of AD, where factors, such as age, gender, mental, and physiological condition, are involved and may be interrelated.

In summary, PRL could promote different effects in NDs depending on gender. In this regard, gender differences are observed in these pathologies, indeed, the incidence rate of AD in women is higher than in men [81]. However, Parkinson's disease (PD) is more prevalent in males than in females [82, 83]. Thus, it is necessary to further explore the neuroprotective role of PRL in both sexes with aging.

6.2 Prolactin and its role in Parkinson's disease

PD is one of the most common neurodegenerative disorders and is a pathology characterized by degeneration of dopaminergic neurons in the substantia nigra pars compacta of the midbrain. Its molecular features are the presence of misfolded alpha-synuclein protein as a cytoplasmic inclusion, named Lewy bodies, in neurons. Genetic factors related to mutation in genes, such as *LRRK2* or *parkin*, have been reported in a small percentage of PD patients [84–87].

Many reports indicate the risk of developing PD is higher in men than in women [82, 83]. Hormone actions, such as estrogen on dopaminergic neuron degeneration, as neuroprotective agents in PD have been widely discussed [88, 89]. Extensive reviews of estrogen as a neuroprotective hormone in PD have been made [90, 91]. Additionally, a study performed in men with PD confirmed increased PRL levels compared to the controls [83]. Thus, PRL probably has different effects on neurodegenerative diseases depending on gender. Thus, the question of whether other hormones related to neuroprotection, such as PRL, have a similar effect in PD opens new avenues for its study. Here, we discussed the role of PRL in PD.

Since PRL secretion is mostly regulated by the dopaminergic pathway [17, 92], many of the pioneer studies were focused on elucidating the relationship between PRL and PD in terms of their interaction with drugs used in PD treatments. For example, Eisler et al. [93] measured PRL and TRH serum levels in parkinsonian patients. Interestingly, PRL and the TRH-induced rise in PRL were normal in patients with PD, whereas levodopa (L-dopa) and carbidopa treatment suppressed PRL concentration in PD patients. These results show how dopaminergic control is in its prime regulation. However, dopaminergic control of PRL in patients with NDs is more complex.

Plasma PRL levels were examined in subjects with PD during the night. Additionally, sleep was assessed to determine the impact of PRL on PD development. The authors reported that plasma PRL levels decreased compared to the controls. Interestingly, these plasma PRL concentrations showed a similar secretion pattern observed in Huntington's patients [94]. Patients with PD associated with major depression and nondepressed Parkinsonians were examined, and PRL and cortisol responses to treatment with fenfluramine (a serotonin-releasing agent) were measured. PRL levels were reduced in patients with PD relative to the controls. Interestingly, PRL was lower in PD patients with major depression compared with the nondepressed patients [95]. Similarly, plasma PRL levels increased with Madopar administration (a combination of L-dopa and benserazide) [96].

Based on the above studies, there are remarkable changes in PRL levels during the progression of PD pathology in response to the conditions of this ND, such as treatment and severity level, which could explain the discrepancies between studies. For example, levels of sex hormones, such as estradiol, testosterone, and PRL, correlated with improvement in quality of life in a study performed in male PD patients.

Surprisingly, PRL levels were significantly increased in the PD group. This suggests a possible involvement of PRL in PD; however, future research is still required to elucidate the role of PRL in PD. As the authors mentioned, a limitation of their research was that the influence of benserazide or carbidopa on the measurement of PRL levels was not taken in consideration [83].

A recent study to discover an accessible biomarker analyzed more than 200 CSF samples using sensitive mass spectrometry (MS)-based proteomics from two independent cohorts. The authors reported specific proteins deregulated in PD patients *versus* the healthy controls. Interestingly, PRL expression was altered in PD samples and correlated with clinical scores [97]. Despite the limitations of this study, very promising biomarkers to understand and improve PD treatment were identified.

Conversely, studies have reported decreased levels in patients with PD. For example, PRL levels were lower in patients with idiopathic PD (IPD) compared to those with multiple system atrophy [98]. In addition to these results, ovariectomized hemiparkinsonian rats treated with estradiol and L-dopa expressed synaptotagmin IV (Syt IV), a gene highly co-expressed with PRL. The authors reported that in this hemiparkinsonian model, high levels of serum from estradiol promoted the upregulation of Syt IV, and consequently of PRL, whereas L-dopa treatment downregulated Syt IV, but no in PRL expression was reported [99]. Interestingly, estradiol and L-dopa are well-known regulators of PRL secretion from the pituitary gland [17]. Beside, in Holstein steer models, L-dopa treatment promotes decreased PRL levels in CSF samples [100]. These results suggest a PRL dysregulation of the dopaminergic pathway in PD.

It is well-known that dysregulation of PRL and TRH levels in patients with PD might be a consequence of damage in TIDA neurons [101]. PRL is regulated by hypothalamic dopaminergic mechanisms. Interestingly, the main drugs used for PD treatment are dopamine precursors: (L-dopa) dopamine agonists (amantadine, apomorphine, bromocriptine, cabergoline, lisuride, pergolide, pramipexole, ropinirole, and rotigotine), monoamine oxidase inhibitors (selegiline and rasagiline), and catechol-O-methyltransferase (COMT) inhibitors (entacapone and tolcapone). For an extensive review see [101]. Notably, PRL has negative and positive interactions with those drugs; however, more research is required to understand the effects that PRL may have on treatments for PD.

In summary, the involvement of PRL in the progression, diagnosis, and development of PD is not fully understood since plasma studies on PRL levels are inconclusive. Therefore, understanding the role of PRL in PD might be useful for the design of therapies to improve the quality of life of patients with PD.

6.3 Evidence of prolactin involvement in Huntington's disease

Huntington's disease (HD) also known as Huntington's chorea is a chronic, progressive, neurodegenerative, and autosomal inherited disorder that severely affects the basal ganglia. HD is a consequence of an extension in a polymorphic trinucleotide repeat of cytosine-adenine-guanine, which is responsible for encoding glutamine. This abnormality is located in exon 1 of the N-terminal coding region of the huntingtin (HTT) [102–104].

The relationship between PRL and HD has been studied for many years [105]. One study showed that patients with HD have low basal and impaired PRL serum levels in response to both, chlorpromazine, and TRH. Another study analyzed basal concentrations of PRL in patients with HD *versus* control subjects and found no significant differences between groups [106]. Durso et al. [107, 108] observed that females with HD had elevated plasma GH levels, in contrast, PRL plasma concentrations in HD patients did not differ from the control [109]. Similarly, PRL serum levels did not increase in HD patients after apomorphine (a dopamine agonist) and muscimol (a GABA agonist) treatments [108].

Conversely, medication-free patients with early-stage HD showed an insignificant increase in PRL serum levels [110]. This could be explained by the alterations in hypothalamic–pituitary dopamine signaling observed in HD and the loss of pituitary D2 receptor expression [111].

Moreover, PRL and other hormones were analyzed in HD and pre-manifest patients. Interestingly, significantly reduced PRL levels were reported in both pre-manifest and HD patients, suggesting that HD patients have an early dysfunction of the hypothalamic-pituitary system since changes in basal PRL levels are detectable early in pre-manifest HD subjects [112]. Concerning changes in PRL levels related to HD development, a study performed in stage II/III HD subjects *versus* healthy controls showed no significant difference in PRL levels between groups [113]. Thus, the role of PRL in HD is still unclear.

Finally, a recent meta-analysis aimed to highlight the possible relation between PRL serum levels and its role in ND development and demonstrated that patients with NDs, specifically in AD and PD, did not have significantly higher serum PRL levels compared with healthy controls; however, in patients with HD, serum PRL levels increased *versus* controls. Nevertheless, due to the heterogeneity among these studies, a subsequent subgroup analysis was performed and indicated that serum PRL levels were higher in the youngest subgroup (<45 years) as observed in a cohort study in Asia and America. Interestingly, the gender subgroup did not show a significant difference in serum PRL levels [109]. Thus, several factors might mediate the diagnosis, progression, and treatment of NDs. Further studies are needed to understand the possible role of PRL as a protective hormone in these complex diseases.

7. The role of prolactin in neuroprotection in the hippocampus

Although few, there are reports indicating an important role of PRL in neuroprotection against excitotoxic damage, specifically in the hippocampus (a brain region that is widely affected due to its large number of glutamatergic receptors) [114, 115]. In postischemic lesions, PRL administration induced the expression of the glial fibrillary acidic protein, promoting astrogliosis [116]. Conversely, after inflicting hypoxic-ischemic injury in ischemia reperfusion by carotid artery occlusion rat model, increased PRLR mRNA and protein were observed in microglia 5 days after injury. This result suggests that PRL may have an important role in inducing astrocytosis [117]. This hints at the additional action that PRL may have in promoting the activation of astrocytes, which ultimately protect neurons. More research is required to elucidate the relation between PRL and astrocyte activation.

Interestingly, a similar protective function was noted after high-dose PRL was administered in rats in global cerebral ischemia induced by bilateral common carotid occlusion. PRL decreased cerebral infarction volume and edema associated with a significant reduction in neurotransmitters, particularly, gamma-aminobutyric acid, Glu, and calcium concentrations [118]. These observations suggest that PRL may restore both physiological and biochemical parameters in the damaged brain tissue. Hence, PRL is a promising molecule in the mitigation of cerebral ischemic damage.

As noted above, PRL mitigates neuronal damage caused by Glu- or KA-induced excitotoxicity, and interestingly, KA administration has been used extensively in rat models of epilepsy. Experiments using varying routes of KA administration, either by IP or ICV, and administering a single dose of PRL via IP, have shown protection of rat hippocampal neuronal density in CA1, CA, and CA4 areas [119–121]. These studies suggest that PRL confers neuroprotection against excitotoxicity by KA. Given that KA is a model of epilepsy, and that PRL mitigates neuronal damage by KA, it may be involved in the mitigation of diseases, such as epilepsy. However, further studies are needed to establish the key molecular mechanisms of PRL in the context of epilepsy. Finally, a recent study about the description of transcriptomic effects by PRL administration in the hippocampus of female rats revealed novel complex gene network interactions induced by PRL, with new functions, such as glial differentiation, axogenesis, synaptic transmission, postsynaptic potential, and neuronal and glial migration [15]. This evidence suggests that PRL is a hormone of interest in neuronal and protective processes.

In summary, prolactin, in addition to lactation, has more than 300 functions and has a significant involvement in the CNS, such as neurogenesis, remyelination, and particularly neuroprotection against excitotoxicity. Although little is known, signaling pathways, such as PI3K/AKT, induction of survival genes, and attenuation of intracellular calcium are the possible mechanisms to explain PRL-induced neuroprotection against excitotoxicity. This neuronal damage mechanism is observed in NDs. Interestingly, PRL plays an important role as a biomarker for some NDs but is also considered a promising molecule for diagnosis. Further, studies are needed to understand the regulation of PRL in NDs, as well as to explore the neuroprotective properties of PRL as a target to develop new treatments and therapies.

8. Conclusion

One of the main characteristics of NDs is excitotoxicity. Thus, it is necessary to further investigate the molecular mechanisms underlying excitotoxicity to prevent neuronal damage or death. Then, elucidating how molecules exert neuroprotective functions and identifying new molecules that exert neuroprotection is mandatory. Accordingly, in this chapter, we described PRL as an important tool to mitigate or prevent neuronal damage in NDs. The study of PRL and its role in NDs opens new avenues for the development of new therapy and treatment strategies for neuroprotection.

Acknowledgements

Gladys Molina-Salinas is a doctoral student from the Programa de Doctorado en Ciencias Biomédicas, Universidad Nacional Autónoma de México (UNAM) and has received CONAHCYT fellowship 892106. This study was supported by grants from PAPIIT IN228420. Dr. Marco Cerbon received a financial support for sabbatical studies from PASPA-DGAPA UNAM.

Conflict of interests

The authors declare that they have no known competing financial interests or personal relationships that could have appeared to influence the data reported in this chapter.

Author details

Gladys Molina-Salinas, Valeria Rodríguez-Chávez and Marco Cerbón*
Faculty of Chemistry, National Autonomous University of Mexico (UNAM), Mexico City, Mexico

*Address all correspondence to: mcerbon85@yahoo.com

References

[1] Rodriguez-Chavez V, Moran J, Molina-Salinas G, et al. Participation of glutamatergic ionotropic receptors in Excitotoxicity: The neuroprotective role of prolactin. Neuroscience. 2021;**461**:180-193. DOI: 10.1016/j.neuroscience.2021.02.027

[2] Armada-Moreira A, Gomes JI, Pina CC, et al. Going the extra (synaptic) mile: Excitotoxicity as the road toward neurodegenerative diseases. Frontiers in Cellular Neuroscience. 2020;**14**:90. DOI: 10.3389/fncel.2020.00090

[3] Mehta A, Prabhakar M, Kumar P, et al. Excitotoxicity: Bridge to various triggers in neurodegenerative disorders. European Journal of Pharmacology. 2013;**698**:6-18. DOI: 10.1016/j.ejphar.2012.10.032

[4] Choi DW. Excitotoxicity: Still hammering the ischemic brain in 2020. Frontiers in Neuroscience. 2020;**14**:579953. DOI: 10.3389/fnins.2020.579953

[5] Avila J, Llorens-Martín M, Pallas-Bazarra N, et al. Cognitive decline in neuronal aging and Alzheimer's disease: Role of NMDA receptors and associated proteins. Frontiers in Neuroscience. 2017;**11**:626. DOI: 10.3389/fnins.2017.00626

[6] Bano D, Ankarcrona M. Beyond the critical point: An overview of excitotoxicity, calcium overload and the downstream consequences. Neuroscience Letters. 2018;**663**:79-85. DOI: 10.1016/j.neulet.2017.08.048

[7] Lewerenz J, Maher P. Chronic glutamate toxicity in neurodegenerative diseases—What is the evidence? Frontiers in Neuroscience. 2015;**9**:1-20. DOI: 10.3389/fnins.2015.00469

[8] Brini M, Calì T, Ottolini D, et al. Neuronal calcium signaling: Function and dysfunction. Cellular and Molecular Life Sciences. 2014;**71**:2787-2814. DOI: 10.1007/s00018-013-1550-7

[9] Hara MR, Snyder SH. Cell signaling and neuronal death. Annual Review of Pharmacology and Toxicology. 2007;**47**:117-141. DOI: 10.1146/annurev.pharmtox.47.120505.105311

[10] Pluta R, Ułamek-Kozioł M, Czuczwar SJ. Neuroprotective and neurological/cognitive enhancement effects of curcumin after brain ischemia injury with alzheimer's disease phenotype. International Journal of Molecular Sciences. 2018;**19**:1-16. DOI: 10.3390/ijms19124002

[11] Ambrogini P, Torquato P, Bartolini D, et al. Excitotoxicity, neuroinflammation and oxidant stress as molecular bases of epileptogenesis and epilepsy-derived neurodegeneration: The role of vitamin E. Biochimica et Biophysica Acta (BBA)—Molecular Basis of Disease. 2019;**1865**:1098-1112. DOI: 10.1016/j.bbadis.2019.01.026

[12] Vanoye-Carlo A, Morales T, Ramos E, et al. Neuroprotective effects of lactation against kainic acid treatment in the dorsal hippocampus of the rat. Hormones and Behavior. 2008;**53**:112-123. DOI: 10.1016/j.yhbeh.2007.09.004

[13] Vergara-Castañeda E, Grattan DR, Pasantes-Morales H, et al. Prolactin mediates neuroprotection against excitotoxicity in primary cell cultures of hippocampal neurons via its receptor. Brain Research. 2016;**1636**:193-199. DOI: 10.1016/j.brainres.2016.02.011

[14] Rivero-Segura NA, Flores-Soto E, De La Cadena SG, et al. Prolactin-induced

neuroprotection against glutamate excitotoxicity is mediated by the reduction of [Ca2+]i overload and NF-κB activation. PLoS One. 2017;**12**:1-16. DOI: 10.1371/journal.pone.0176910

[15] Cabrera-Reyes EA, Vanoye–Carlo A, Rodríguez-Dorantes M, et al. Transcriptomic analysis reveals new hippocampal gene networks induced by prolactin. Scientific Reports. 2019;**9**:1-12. DOI: 10.1038/s41598-019-50228-7

[16] Molina-Salinas G, Rivero-Segura NA, Cabrera-Reyes EA, et al. Decoding signaling pathways involved in prolactin-induced neuroprotection: A review. Frontiers in Neuroendocrinology. 2021;**61**:100913. DOI: 10.1016/j.yfrne.2021.100913

[17] Freeman ME, Kanyicska LA, Lerant A, et al. Prolactin: Structure , function , and regulation of secretion. American Physiological Society. 2000;**80**:1523-1631. DOI: 10.1152/physrev.2000.80.4.1523

[18] Cabrera-Reyes EA, Limón-Morales O, Rivero-Segura NA, et al. Prolactin function and putative expression in the brain. Endocrine. 2017;**57**:199-213. DOI: 10.1007/s12020-017-1346-x

[19] Ben-Jonathan N, LaPensee CR, LaPensee EW. What can we learn from rodents about prolactin in humans? Endocrine Reviews. 2008;**29**:1-41. DOI: 10.1210/er.2007-0017

[20] Patil MJ, Henry MA, Akopian AN. Prolactin receptor in regulation of neuronal excitability and channels. Channels. 2014;**8**:193-202. DOI: 10.4161/chan.28946

[21] Bernard V, Young J, Chanson P, et al. New insights in prolactin: Pathological implications. Nature Reviews. Endocrinology. 2015;**11**:265-275. DOI: 10.1038/nrendo.2015.36

[22] Bernard V, Young J, Binart N. Prolactin—A pleiotropic factor in health and disease. Nature Reviews. Endocrinology. 2019;**15**:356-365. DOI: 10.1038/s41574-019-0194-6

[23] Grattan DR, Kokay IC. Prolactin: A pleiotropic neuroendocrine hormone. Journal of Neuroendocrinology. 2008;**20**:752-763. DOI: 10.1111/j.1365-2826.2008.01736.x

[24] Binart N. Prolactin and pregnancy in mice and humans. Annales d'endocrinologie. 2016;**77**:126-127. DOI: 10.1016/j.ando.2016.04.008

[25] Marano RJ, Ben-Jonathan N. Minireview: Extrapituitary prolactin: An update on the distribution, regulation, and functions. Molecular Endocrinology. 2014;**28**:622-633. DOI: 10.1210/me.2013-1349

[26] Costanza M, Pedotti R. Prolactin: Friend or foe in central nervous system autoimmune inflammation? International Journal of Molecular Sciences. 2016;**17**:2012-2016. DOI: 10.3390/ijms17122026

[27] Costa-Brito AR, Gonçalves I, Santos CRA. The brain as a source and a target of prolactin in mammals. Neural Regeneration Research. 2022;**17**:1695-1702. DOI: 10.4103/1673-5374.332124

[28] Carretero J, Sánchez-Robledo V, Carretero-Hernández M, et al. Prolactin system in the hippocampus. Cell and Tissue Research. 2019;**375**:193-199. DOI: 10.1007/s00441-018-2858-2

[29] Gorvin CM. The prolactin receptor: Diverse and emerging roles in pathophysiology. Journal of Clinical & Translational Endocrinology. 2015;**2**:85-91. DOI: 10.1016/j.jcte.2015.05.001

[30] Molina-Salinas G, Rodríguez-Chávez V, Langley E, et al.

Prolactin-induced neuroprotection against excitotoxicity is mediated via PI3K/AKT and GSK3β/NF-κB in primary cultures of hippocampal neurons. Peptides. 2023;**166**:171037. DOI: 10.1016/j.peptides.2023.171037

[31] Sangeeta Devi Y, Halperin J. Reproductive actions of prolactin mediated through short and long receptor isoforms. Molecular and Cellular Endocrinology. 2014;**382**:400-410. DOI: 10.1016/j.mce.2013.09.016

[32] Torner L, Neumann ID. The brain prolactin system: Involvement in stress response adaptations in lactation. Stress. 2002;**5**:249-257. DOI: 10.1080/1025389021000048638

[33] Horseman ND, Gregerson KA. Prolactin actions. Journal of Molecular Endocrinology. 2013;**19**:95-106. DOI: 10.1530/JME-13-0220

[34] Bole-Feysot C, Goffin V, Edery M, et al. Prolactin (PRL) and its receptor: Actions, signal transduction pathways and phenotypes observed in PRL receptor knockout mice. Endocrine Reviews. 1998;**19**:225-268. DOI: 10.1210/edrv.19.3.0334

[35] Borba VV, Zandman-Goddard G, Shoenfeld Y. Prolactin and autoimmunity: The hormone as an inflammatory cytokine. Best Practice & Research. Clinical Endocrinology & Metabolism. 2019;**33**:101324. DOI: 10.1016/j.beem.2019.101324

[36] Torner L. Actions of prolactin in the brain: From physiological adaptations to stress and neurogenesis to psychopathology. Frontiers in Endocrinology. 2016;**7**(25):1-6. DOI: 10.3389/fendo.2016.0002

[37] Larsen CM, Grattan DR. Prolactin-induced mitogenesis in the subventricular zone of the maternal brain during early pregnancy is essential for normal postpartum behavioral responses in the mother. Endocrinology. 2010;**151**:3805-3814. DOI: 10.1210/en.2009-1385

[38] Walker TL, Vukovic J, Koudijs MM, et al. Prolactin stimulates precursor cells in the adult mouse hippocampus. PLoS One. 2012;**7**:1-11. DOI: 10.1371/journal.pone.0044371

[39] Rivero-Segura NA, Coronado-Mares MI, Rincón-Heredia R, et al. Prolactin prevents mitochondrial dysfunction induced by glutamate excitotoxicity in hippocampal neurons. Neuroscience Letters. 2019;**701**:58-64. DOI: 10.1016/j.neulet.2019.02.027

[40] Olney JW, Price MT, Samson L, et al. The role of specific ions in glutamate neurotoxicity. Neuroscience Letters. 1986;**65**:65-71. DOI: 10.1016/0304-3940(86)90121-7

[41] Choi DW. Excitotoxic cell death. Journal of Neurobiology. 1992;**23**:1261-1276. DOI: 10.1002/neu.480230915

[42] Dong X, Wang Y, Qin Z. Molecular mechanisms of excitotoxicity and their relevance to pathogenesis of neurodegenerative diseases. Acta Pharmacologica Sinica. 2009;**30**:379-387. DOI: 10.1038/aps.2009.24

[43] Reiner A, Levitz J. Glutamatergic signaling in the central nervous system: Ionotropic and metabotropic receptors in concert. Neuron. 2018;**98**:1080-1098. DOI: 10.1016/j.neuron.2018.05.018

[44] Hansen KB, Wollmuth LP, Bowie D, et al. Structure, function, and pharmacology of glutamate receptor ion channels. Pharmacological Reviews. 2021;**73**:298-487. DOI: 10.1124/pharmrev.120.000131

[45] Gross A, Katz SG. Non-apoptotic functions of BCL-2 family proteins. Cell Death and Differentiation. 2017;**24**:1348-1358. DOI: 10.1038/cdd.2017.22

[46] Zamani M, Hassanshahi J, Soleimani M, et al. Neuroprotective effect of olive oil in the hippocampus CA1 neurons following ischemia: Reperfusion in mice. Journal of Neurosciences in Rural Practice. 2013;**4**:164-170. DOI: 10.4103/0976-3147.112753

[47] Zheng X-Y, Zhang H-L, Luo Q, et al. Kainic acid-induced neurodegenerative model: Potentials and limitations. Journal of Biomedicine & Biotechnology. 2011;**2011**:457079. DOI: 10.1155/2011/457079

[48] Torner L, Karg S, Blume A, et al. Prolactin prevents chronic stress-induced decrease of adult hippocampal neurogenesis and promotes neuronal fate. The Journal of Neuroscience. 2009;**29**:1826-1833. DOI: 10.1523/JNEUROSCI.3178-08.2009

[49] Rodríguez-Chávez V, Flores-Soto E, Molina-Salinas G, et al. Prolactin reduces the kainic acid-induced increase in intracellular Ca2+ concentration, leading to neuroprotection of hippocampal neurons. Neuroscience Letters. 2023;**810**:137344. DOI: 10.1016/j.neulet.2023.137344

[50] Bredesen DE, Rao RV, Mehlen P. Cell death in the nervous system. Nature. 2006;**443**:796-802. DOI: 10.1038/nature05293

[51] Glass CK, Saijo K, Winner B, et al. Mechanisms underlying inflammation in neurodegeneration. Cell. 2010;**140**:918-934. DOI: 10.1016/j.cell.2010.02.016

[52] Ross CA, Poirier MA. Protein aggregation and neurodegenerative disease. Nature Medicine. 2004;**10**:S10. DOI: 10.1038/nm1066

[53] Dutta RTB. Mechanisms of neuronal dysfunction and degeneration in multiple sclerosis. Progress in Neurobiology. 2011;**93**:1-12. DOI: 10.1016/j.pneurobio.2010.09.005

[54] Matías-Guiu JA, Oreja-Guevara C, Cabrera-Martín MN, et al. Amyloid proteins and their role in multiple sclerosis. Considerations in the use of amyloid-PET imaging. Frontiers in Neurology. 2016;**7**:1-7. DOI: 10.3389/fneur.2016.00053

[55] Hynd MR, Scott HL, Dodd PR. Glutamate-mediated excitotoxicity and neurodegeneration in Alzheimer's disease. Neurochemistry International. 2004;**45**:583-595. DOI: 10.1016/j.neuint.2004.03.007

[56] Kovacs GG. Molecular pathological classification of neurodegenerative diseases: Turning towards precision medicine. International Journal of Molecular Sciences. 2016;**17**:2-89. DOI: 10.3390/ijms17020189

[57] Kovacs GG. Concepts and classification of neurodegenerative diseases. Handbook of Clinical Neurology. 2017;**145**:301-307. DOI: 10.1016/B978-0-12-802395-2.00021-3

[58] Dugger BN, Dickson DW. Pathology of neurodegenerative diseases. Cold Spring Harbor Perspectives in Biology. 2017;**9**:1-22. DOI: 10.1101/cshperspect.a028035

[59] Hardy J, Duff K, Hardy KG, et al. Genetic dissection of Alzheimer's disease and related dementias: Amyloid and its relationship to tau. Nature Neuroscience. 1998;**1**:355-358. DOI: 10.1038/1565

[60] Franceschi M, Perego L, Ferini-Strambi L, et al. Neuroendocrinological function in Alzheimer's disease. Neuroendocrinology. 1988;**48**:367-370. DOI: 10.1159/000125036

[61] Duc Nguyen H, Pal YB, Hoang NHM, et al. Prolactin and its altered action in Alzheimer's disease and Parkinson's disease. Neuroendocrinology. 2022;**112**:427-445. DOI: 10.1159/000517798

[62] House A, Jones J. Increased response of serum prolactin to metoclopramide in senile dementia of Alzheimer type. International Journal of Geriatric Psychiatry. 1989;**4**:279-282. DOI: 10.1002/gps.930040506

[63] Bille A, Olafsson K, Jensen HV, et al. Prolactin responses to thyrotropin-releasing hormone in multi-infarct dementia and senile dementia of the Alzheimer type. Acta Psychiatrica Scandinavica. 1991;**83**:321-323. DOI: 10.1111/j.1600-0447.1991.tb05548.x

[64] Pedrós I, Petrov D, Artiach G, et al. Adipokine pathways are altered in hippocampus of an experimental mouse model of Alzheimer's disease. The Journal of Nutrition, Health & Aging. 2015;**19**:403-412. DOI: 10.1007/s12603-014-0574-5

[65] Kitagishi Y, Matsuda S. Diets involved in PPAR and PI3K/AKT/PTEN pathway may contribute to neuroprotection in a traumatic brain injury. Alzheimer's Research and Therapy. 2013;**5**:1. DOI: 10.1186/alzrt208

[66] Matsuda S, Nakagawa Y, Tsuji A, et al. Implications of PI3K/AKT/PTEN signaling on superoxide Dismutases expression and in the pathogenesis of Alzheimer's disease. Diseases. 2018;**6**:1-13. DOI: 10.3390/diseases6020028

[67] Plotnikov A, Li Y, Tran TH, et al. Oncogene-mediated inhibition of glycogen synthase kinase 3 beta impairs degradation of prolactin receptor. Cancer Research. 2008;**68**:1354-1361. DOI: 10.1158/0008-5472.CAN-07-6094

[68] Muñoz-Mayorga D, Guerra-Araiza C, Torner L, et al. Tau phosphorylation in female neurodegeneration: Role of estrogens, progesterone, and prolactin. Frontiers in Endocrinology. 2018;**9**:1-8. DOI: 10.3389/fendo.2018.00133

[69] Steinmetz D, Ramos E, Campbell SN, et al. Reproductive stage and modulation of stress-induced tau phosphorylation in female rats. Journal of Neuroendocrinology. 2015;**27**:827-834. DOI: 10.1111/jne.12323

[70] Grattan DR. The hypothalamo-prolactin axis. The Journal of Endocrinology. 2015;**226**:101-122. DOI: 10.1530/JOE-15-0213

[71] Dudas B, Merchenthaler I. Thyrotropin-releasing hormone axonal varicosities appear to innervate dopaminergic neurons in the human hypothalamus. Brain Structure & Function. 2020;**225**:2193-2201. DOI: 10.1007/s00429-020-02120-8

[72] Luo L, Stopa EG. Thyrotropin releasing hormone inhibits tau phosphorylation by dual signaling pathways in hippocampal neurons. Journal of Alzheimer's Disease. 2004;**6**:527-536. DOI: 10.3233/jad-2004-6510

[73] van Osch LADM, Hogervorst E, Combrinck M, et al. Low thyroid-stimulating hormone as an independent risk factor for Alzheimer disease. Neurology. 2004;**62**:1967-1971. DOI: 10.1212/01.wnl.0000128134.84230.9f

[74] Labudova O, Cairns N, Koeck T, et al. Thyroid stimulating hormone—Receptor overexpression in brain of patients with down syndrome and Alzheimer's disease. Life Sciences. 1999;**64**:1037-1044. DOI: 10.1016/s0024-3205(99)00030-2

[75] Daimon CM, Chirdon P, Maudsley S, et al. The role of thyrotropin releasing hormone in aging and neurodegenerative diseases. American Journal of Alzheimer's Disease (Columbia). 2013;**1**:10.7726. DOI: 10.7726/ajad.2013.1003

[76] Tan ZS, Beiser A, Vasan RS, et al. Thyroid function and the risk of Alzheimer disease: The Framingham study. Archives of Internal Medicine. 2008;**168**:1514-1520. DOI: 10.1001/archinte.168.14.1514

[77] Zetterberg H, Bendlin BB. Biomarkers for Alzheimer's disease—Preparing for a new era of disease-modifying therapies. Molecular Psychiatry. 2021;**26**:296-308. DOI: 10.1038/s41380-020-0721-9

[78] Leung YY, Toledo JB, Nefedov A, et al. Identifying amyloid pathology-related cerebrospinal fluid biomarkers for Alzheimer's disease in a multicohort study. Alzheimer's & Dementia: Diagnosis, Assessment & Disease Monitoring. 2015;**1**:339-348. DOI: 10.1016/j.dadm.2015.06.008

[79] Zverova M, Kitzlerova E, Fisar Z, et al. Interplay between the APOE genotype and possible plasma biomarkers in Alzheimer's disease. Current Alzheimer Research. 2018;**15**:938-950. DOI: 10.2174/1567205015666180601090533

[80] Tariot PN, Upadhyaya A, Sunderland T, et al. Physiologic and neuroendocrine responses to intravenous naloxone in subjects with Alzheimer's disease and age-matched controls. Biological Psychiatry. 1999;**46**:412-419. DOI: 10.1016/s0006-3223(98)00329-1

[81] Beama CR, Kaneshiro C, Jang JY, Reynolds CA, Pedersen NL, Gatz M. Differences between women and men in incidence rates of dementia and Alzheimer's disease. Journal of Alzheimer's Disease. 2018;**64**:1077-1083. DOI: 10.3233/JAD-180141

[82] Riedel O, Bitters D, Amann U, et al. Estimating the prevalence of Parkinson's disease (PD) and proportions of patients with associated dementia and depression among the older adults based on secondary claims data. International Journal of Geriatric Psychiatry. 2016;**31**:938-943. DOI: 10.1002/gps.4414

[83] Nitkowska M, Tomasiuk R, Czyzyk M, et al. Prolactin and sex hormones levels in males with Parkinson's disease. Acta Neurologica Scandinavica. 2015;**131**:411-416. DOI: 10.1111/ane.12334

[84] Matilla-Dueñas A, Corral-Juan M, Rodríguez-Palmero Seuma A, et al. Rare neurodegenerative diseases: Clinical and genetic update. Advances in experimental medicine and biology. Advances in Experimental Medicine and Biology. 2017;**1031**:443-496. DOI: 10.1007/978-3-319-67144-4_25

[85] Heller J, Dogan I, Schulz JB, et al. Evidence for gender differences in cognition, emotion and quality of life in Parkinson's disease? Aging and Disease. 2014;**5**:63-75. DOI: 10.14366/AD.2014.050063

[86] Hayes MT. Parkinson's disease and parkinsonism. The American Journal of Medicine. 2019;**132**:802-807. DOI: 10.1016/j.amjmed.2019.03.001

[87] Cerri S, Mus L, Blandini F. Parkinson's disease in women and men: What's the difference? Journal of Parkinson's Disease. 2019;**9**:501-515. DOI: 10.3233/JPD-191683

[88] Solla P, Cannas A, Ibba FC, et al. Gender differences in motor and non-motor symptoms among Sardinian

patients with Parkinson's disease. Journal of the Neurological Sciences. 2012;**323**:33-39. DOI: 10.1016/j.jns.2012.07.026

[89] Liu B, Dluzen DE. Oestrogen and nigrostriatal dopaminergic neurodegeneration: Animal models and clinical reports of Parkinson's disease. Clinical and Experimental Pharmacology & Physiology. 2007;**34**:555-565. DOI: 10.1111/j.1440-1681.2007.04616.x

[90] Saunders-Pullman R, Gordon-Elliott J, Parides M, et al. The effect of estrogen replacement on early Parkinson's disease. Neurology. 1999;**52**:1417-1421. DOI: 10.1212/wnl.52.7.1417 DOI: 10.1212/wnl.52.7.1417

[91] Członkowska A, Ciesielska A, Gromadzka G, et al. Gender differences in neurological disease: Role of estrogens and cytokines. Endocrine. 2006;**29**:243-256. DOI: 10.1385/ENDO:29:2:243

[92] Gustafson P, Kokay I, Sapsford T, et al. Prolactin regulation of the HPA axis is not mediated by a direct action upon CRH neurons: Evidence from the rat and mouse. Brain Structure & Function. 2017;**222**:3191-3204. DOI: 10.1007/s00429-017-1395-1

[93] Eisler T, Thorner MO, MacLeod RM, et al. Prolactin secretion in Parkinson disease. Neurology. 1981;**31**:1356-1359. DOI: 10.1212/wnl.31.10.1356

[94] Murri L, Iudice A, Muratorio A, et al. Spontaneous nocturnal plasma prolactin and growth hormone secretion in patients with Parkinson's disease and Huntington's chorea. European Neurology. 1980;**19**:198-206. DOI: 10.1159/000115147

[95] Kostić VS, Lecić D, Doder M, et al. Prolactin and cortisol responses to fenfluramine in Parkinson's disease. Biological Psychiatry. 1996;**40**:769-775. DOI: 10.1016/0006-3223(95)00496-3

[96] Martinez-Campos A, Giovannini P, Parati E, et al. Growth hormone and prolactin stimulation by Madopar in Parkinson's disease. Journal of Neurology, Neurosurgery, and Psychiatry. 1981;**44**:1116-1123. DOI: 10.1136/jnnp.44.12.1116

[97] Karayel O, Virreira Winter S, Padmanabhan S, et al. Proteome profiling of cerebrospinal fluid reveals biomarker candidates for Parkinson's disease. Cell Reports Medicine. 2022;**3**:100661. DOI: 10.1016/j.xcrm.2022.100661

[98] Winkler AS, Landau S, Chaudhuri KR. Serum prolactin levels in Parkinson's disease and multiple system atrophy. Clinical Autonomic Research. 2002;**12**:393-398. DOI: 10.1007/s10286-002-0025-y

[99] Zorovic M, Kolmančič K, Živin M. Effects of L-dopa on expression of prolactin and synaptotagmin IV in 17-beta-estradiol-induced prolactinomas of ovariectomized hemiparkinsonian rats. Bosnian Journal of Basic Medical Sciences. 2021;**21**:702-711. DOI: 10.17305/bjbms.2021.5491

[100] Kasuya E, Yayou K, Sutoh M. L-DOPA attenuates prolactin secretion in response to isolation stress in Holstein steers. Animal Science Journal. 2013;**84**:562-568. DOI: 10.1111/asj.12037

[101] Cacabelos R. Parkinson's disease: From pathogenesis to pharmacogenomics. International Journal of Molecular Sciences. 2017;**18**:533-551. DOI: 10.3390/ijms18030551

[102] Müller T. Investigational agents for the management of Huntington's disease. Expert Opinion on

Investigational Drugs. 2017;**26**:175-185. DOI: 10.1080/13543784.2017.1270266

[103] Paulsen JS, Long JD, Ross CA, et al. Prediction of manifest Huntington's disease with clinical and imaging measures: A prospective observational study. Lancet Neurology. 2014;**13**:1193-1201. DOI: 10.1016/S1474-4422(14)70238-8

[104] Kim A, Lalonde K, Truesdell A, et al. New avenues for the treatment of Huntington's disease. International Journal of Molecular Sciences. 2021;**22**:8363. DOI: 10.3390/ijms22168363

[105] Hayden MR, Vinik AI, Paul M, et al. Impaired prolactin release in Huntington's chorea. Evidence for dopaminergic excess. Lancet. 1977;**2**:423-426. DOI: 10.1016/s0140-6736(77)90608-0

[106] Chalmers RJ, Johnson RH, Keogh HJ, et al. Growth hormone and prolactin response to bromocriptine in patients with Huntington's chorea. Journal of Neurology, Neurosurgery, and Psychiatry. 1978;**41**:135-139. DOI: 10.1136/jnnp.41.2.135

[107] Durso R, Tamminga CA, Ruggeri S, et al. Twenty-four hour plasma levels of growth hormone and prolactin in Huntington's disease. Journal of Neurology, Neurosurgery, and Psychiatry. 1983;**46**:1134-1137. DOI: 10.1136/jnnp.46.12.1134

[108] Durso R, Tamminga CA, Denaro A, et al. Plasma growth hormone and prolactin response to dopaminergic GABAmimetic and cholinergic stimulation in Huntington's disease. Neurology. 1983;**33**:1229-1232. DOI: 10.1212/wnl.33.9.1299

[109] Duc Nguyen H, Hoang NMH, Ko M, et al. Association between serum prolactin levels and neurodegenerative diseases: Systematic review and meta-analysis. Neuroimmunomodulation. 2022;**29**:85-96. DOI: 10.1159/000519552

[110] Aziz NA, Pijl H, Frölich M, et al. Altered thyrotropic and lactotropic axes regulation in Huntington's disease. Clinical Endocrinology. 2010;**73**:540-545. DOI: 10.1111/j.1365-2265.2010.03836.x

[111] Björkqvist M, Petersén A, Bacos K, et al. Progressive alterations in the hypothalamic-pituitary-adrenal axis in the R6/2 transgenic mouse model of Huntington's disease. Human Molecular Genetics. 2006;**15**:1713-1721. DOI: 10.1093/hmg/ddl094

[112] Wang R, Ross CA, Cai H, et al. Metabolic and hormonal signatures in pre-manifest and manifest Huntington's disease patients. Frontiers in Physiology. 2014;**5**:231. DOI: 10.3389/fphys.2014.00231

[113] Kalliolia E, Silajdžić E, Nambron R, et al. A 24-hour study of the Hypothalamo-pituitary axes in Huntington's disease. PLoS One. 2015;**10**:e0138848. DOI: 10.1371/journal.pone.0138848

[114] Baude A, Nusser Z, Molnar E, et al. High-resolution immunogold localization of AMPA type glutamate receptor subunits at synaptic and non-synaptic sites in rat hippocampus. Neuroscience. 1995;**69**:1031-1055. DOI: 10.1016/0306-4522(95)00350-r

[115] Wenk GL, Barnes CA. Regional changes in the hippocampal density of AMPA and NMDA receptors across the lifespan of the rat. Brain Research. 2000;**885**:1-5. DOI: 10.1016/s0006-8993(00)02792-x

[116] Anagnostou I, Reyes-Mendoza J, Morales T. Glial cells as mediators of

protective actions of prolactin (PRL) in the CNS. General and Comparative Endocrinology. 2018;**265**:106-110. DOI: 10.1016/j.ygcen.2018.01.024

[117] Möderscheim TAE, Gorba T, Pathipati P, et al. Prolactin is involved in glial responses following a focal injury to the juvenile rat brain. Neuroscience. 2007;**145**:963-973. DOI: 10.1016/j.neuroscience.2006.12.053

[118] Vermani B, Mukherjee S, Kumar G, et al. Prolactin attenuates global cerebral ischemic injury in rat model by conferring neuroprotection. Brain Injury. 2020;**34**:685-693. DOI: 10.1080/02699052.2020.1726466

[119] Cabrera V, Cantú D, Ramos E, et al. Lactation is a natural model of hippocampus neuroprotection against excitotoxicity. Neuroscience Letters. 2009;**461**:136-139. DOI: 10.1016/j.neulet.2009.06.017

[120] Tejadilla D, Cerbón M, Morales T. Prolactin reduces the damaging effects of excitotoxicity in the dorsal hippocampus of the female rat independently of ovarian hormones. Neuroscience. 2010;**169**:1178-1185. DOI: 10.1016/j.neuroscience.2010.05.074

[121] Ortiz-Pérez A, Limón-Morales O, Rojas-Castañeda JC, et al. Prolactin prevents the kainic acid-induced neuronal loss in the rat hippocampus by inducing prolactin receptor and putatively increasing the VGLUT1 overexpression. Neuroscience Letters. 2019;**694**:116-123. DOI: 10.1016/j.neulet.2018.11.052

Chapter 6

Cardioprotection Using Doxorubicin: The Role of Dexrazoxane

Ronald J. Krone, Azim Merchant and Joshua D. Mitchell

Abstract

Doxorubicin is among the most effective chemotherapeutic agents, and is active against a wide variety of cancers. However, it also is highly cardiotoxic so that any effective use of this agent requires a strategy to limit the toxicity. Dexrazoxane is the only drug approved specifically to counter the cardiac toxicity of doxorubicin because of its ability to interfere with the molecular mechanisms causing the cardiac injury. Although other mechanisms, namely iron chelating properties, were originally thought to be responsible for its cardiac protection, recent studies suggest that dexrazoxane's interaction with topoisomerase II, an enzyme important for the function of DNA during mitosis is most likely the major mechanism. While it had been thought that the mechanism of doxorubicin's cardiac toxicity and the mechanism of doxorubicin's tumor effectiveness are different, more recent studies have suggested that some of the most important mechanisms are similar. Because of this uncertainty, dexrazoxane is underutilized in patients where it could be useful. Thus, studies comparing tumor efficacy in patients taking doxorubicin randomized to dexrazoxane comparing progression-free survival and mortality as well as cancer treatment-related cardiac dysfunction (CTRCD) are needed to give oncologists data to support aggressive use of dexrazoxane in their patients.

Keywords: doxorubicin, cardiotoxicity, dexrazoxane, topoisomerase II, cardio-protection, sarcoma

1. Introduction

Doxorubicin, a member of a class of cancer chemotherapeutic agents derived from Streptomyces bacterium, is among the most effective chemotherapeutic agents active against a wide variety of cancers [1, 2], primarily solid tumors (breast, lymphomas, lung [1, 2] and especially sarcomas [3]. It is also effective against leukemias but often in combination with other agents and with more limited dosing. Unfortunately, the development of chemo-resistance and the development of cardiac toxicity limits its widespread applicability. A number of strategies have been developed to limit cardiotoxicity to allow more of the drug to be safely administered. Dexrazoxane is the only drug approved specifically to counter the cardiac toxicity of doxorubicin. Only dexrazoxane is able to directly interfere with the molecular mechanisms causing the cardiac injury. Originally proposed for its iron chelating properties, dexrazoxane more likely acts by inhibiting the effect of doxorubicin on topoisomerase IIB (TOPIIβ), though other mechanisms have also been suggested. While it has been held that the mechanisms of doxorubicin's cardiac toxicity and the mechanism of doxorubicin's tumor effectiveness are different, more recent studies have suggested that some of the most important mechanisms are similar. Because of this uncertainty, additional studies are needed to compare tumor efficacy in patients taking and not taking dexrazoxane to establish whether dexrazoxane, in addition to protecting the heart, does not reduce progression-free survival and increase cancer-related mortality.

2. Mechanism of action of doxorubicin

Doxorubicin kills tumor cells through several unrelated mechanisms (**Figure 1** and **Table 1**). After diffusing into the nucleus, it disrupts many targets: intercalating into DNA and interrupting DNA synthesis, inhibiting RNA synthesis and binding with TOPII, an enzyme essential to the reproduction of DNA, with subsequent DNA damage and induction of apoptosis [2, 4–7]. Doxorubicin's intercalation into DNA ultimately leads to inhibited synthesis of macromolecules. Interaction with TOPII impedes DNA resealing during mitosis and is a major mechanism for

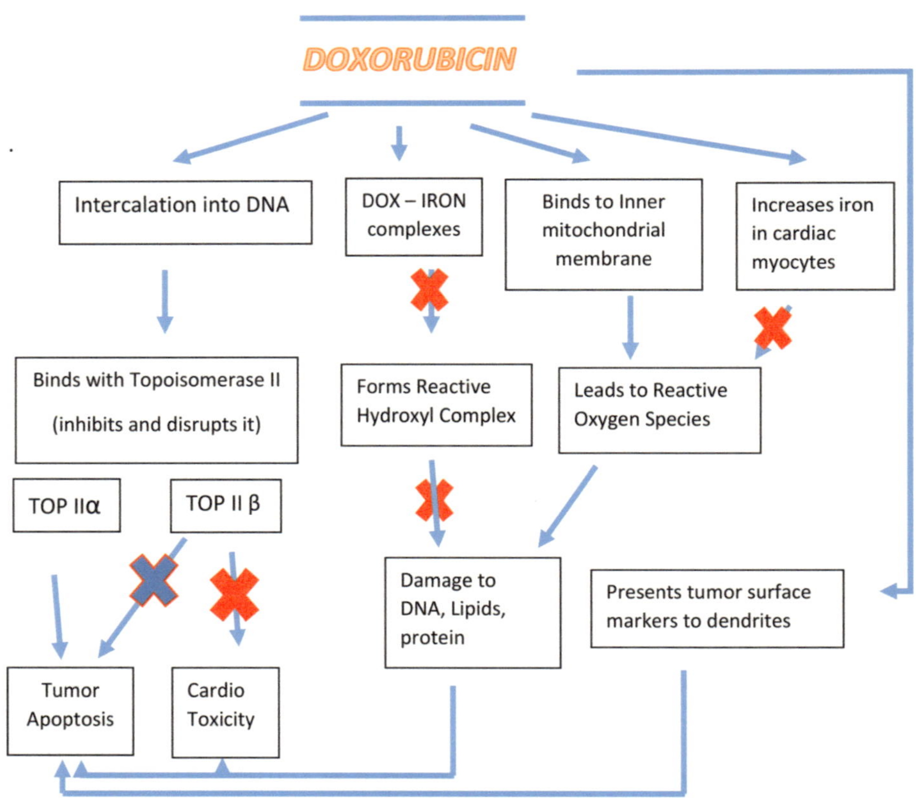

Figure 1.
Diagrammatic representation of the mechanisms of action of doxorubicin. The large red X represents the areas where dexrazoxane blocks the action of doxorubicin on the cardiac myocytes. The blue X marks where dexrazoxane may block the effect of doxorubicin on TOP2α which is the major action in destroying the tumor.

Doxorubicin kills tumor cells through several unrelated mechanisms.
1. DNA in the nucleus intercalates into DNA, and a. interrupts DNA synthesis. b. Inhibits RNA synthesis. c. binds with TOPII with subsequent DNA damage and induction of apoptosis [2, 4–6]. d. leads to inhibited synthesis of macromolecules.
2. Interaction with TOPII impedes DNA resealing during mitosis.
3. Changes the surface markers of the tumor allowing dendritic cells to recognize the tumor-- activating the immune system.
4. Binds to the inner mitochondrial membrane phospholipid and generates (ROS) which damages the cell and leads to apoptosis which exposes tumor proteins activating the immune system [8].
5. Complexes with iron producing reactive hydroxyl radicals with DNA, lipid and protein damage [10].
6. Increases the concentration of iron in cardiac myocytes, producing hydroxyl radicals.
7. Disrupts calcium metabolism, further interfering with cardiac contraction [11].

Table 1.
Mechanisms of action of doxorubicin [2].

tumor destruction as well as cardiac toxicity. Doxorubicin also makes changes in the surface markers of the tumor allowing the dendritic cells to recognize the tumor and activate the immune system by stimulating killer cells and by other less-understood mechanisms. It binds to the inner mitochondrial membrane phospholipid, inhibiting aspects of the electron transporter chain and leading to the generation of reactive oxygen species (ROS) [8]. These molecules damage multiple cellular components such as lipids, proteins and DNA [9] and in severe exposures can lead to apoptosis. Doxorubicin also reacts with iron and the doxorubicin-iron complex catalyzes the conversion of H_2O_2 and O_2 into reactive hydroxyl radicals that also lead to DNA, lipid and protein damage [10]. In addition to these effects on the tumor, anthracyclines can increase the concentration of iron within cardiac myocytes, which contributes to the formation of ROS-producing hydroxyl radicals. Finally, anthracyclines disrupt calcium metabolism, further interfering with cardiac contraction [11].

3. Cardiac toxicity with doxorubicin

Cardiac toxicity manifested as cancer treatment-related cardiac dysfunction (CTRCD) is common with doxorubicin and is dose related [12]. Toxicity to other organs, liver, kidneys and brain can also occur [6]. As early as 1987 Schwartz et al. reported that 16% of patients deemed at high risk for cardiotoxicity because of a high administered doxorubicin dose or a decline in left ventricular (LV) ejection fraction developed congestive failure. Of these, five continued with persistent LV dysfunction and one person died from cardiac failure [13]. An excellent history of the discovery of the toxicity of doxorubicin and the development of strategies to limit the toxicity is discussed by Benjamin and Minotti [14].

Careful monitoring of LV function with advanced imaging strategies to identify the earliest appearance of cardiac toxicity is recommended before severe cardiac dysfunction has developed. This facilitates the initiation of cardioprotective strategies either with dose modification or with cardioprotective medications hopefully before irreversible dysfunction develops [15]. Early treatment of CTRCD allows recovery of function in many patients, which may not happen if treatment is delayed [16].

Strategies of surveillance have been described [17]. This includes baseline evaluation of biomarkers, and especially measures of LV function. Echocardiography is currently recommended with careful measurement of LV ejection fraction using two-dimensional (2D) evaluation using Simpson's rule. The use of echo contrast when images are inadequate is strongly encouraged [15, 18, 19]. Three-dimensional (3D) imaging has been recommended as a technique which may be more reproducible and is being investigated. However, it depends on high-quality imaging which may be less available in the clinical setting than in a research laboratory [20]. Measurement of global longitudinal strain has been promoted as a measure of ventricular function and may identify CTRCD before cardiac dysfunction manifests with the ejection fraction [18, 21, 22]. Other measures of LV function, such as cardiac magnetic resonance imaging can be used when echo images cannot be obtained [15] and offer the advantage of being able to image myocardial abnormalities such as edema or fibrosis. In high-risk patients, imaging usually with every other dose of doxorubicin has been recommended [15].

4. Limiting the cardiac toxicity of doxorubicin

Cardiac toxicity, in the form of a depression of primarily LV function is a major consideration when using doxorubicin. Cardiac toxicity can lead to serious morbidity and even death in persons who otherwise may have survived their cancer. Where doxorubicin is holding the tumor in check but not eliminating it, the development of cardiotoxicity will require stopping the doxorubicin with the likely result that control may be lost over the tumor.

An early approach to reducing doxorubicin cardiotoxicity was to limit the dose to less than 550 mg/M2 [12, 23]. Of course, this has the disadvantage of restricting the use of doxorubicin. Such a strategy is especially problematic if the doxorubicin is controlling the tumor and is the most effective chemotherapeutic option. This is especially true in the management of sarcomas. More recently there have been a large number of controlled studies evaluating drugs which are used in the treatment of heart failure (GDMT) to determine if they can protect against CTRCD from doxorubicin [16, 24–27].

Beta blockers differ in their mechanism of actions, and their effectiveness in this role of protecting against LV depression from chemotherapy varies. Carvedilol a non-selective beta blocker with antioxidant activity [28] and nebivolol a cardioselective beta blocker with antioxidant activity and a nitric oxide donor [29] are somewhat protective but metoprolol [30, 31] did not protect. Enalapril among the ACE inhibitors in an early study was found to be protective [32] but in a larger study with 125 patients showed no effect [31]. The combination of enalapril and carvedilol prevented LV deterioration with doxorubicin. Valsartan [33], telemesartan [34] and candesartan [30] have also been shown protective efficacy.

Spironolactone has been shown to be protective when given simultaneously with doxorubicin [35]. Spironolactone may be a poor choice in breast cancer since it blocks adrenergic hormones. Presumably, eplerenone could be substituted in these patients since it does not affect adrenergic hormones but this has not been studied.

Statins have been explored as a possible cardioprotection agent and an association between statin use and decreased toxicity of anthracyclines has been shown in a meta-analysis [36, 37].

Sodium glucose co-transporter 2 (SGLT-2) inhibitors have more recently been reported to be beneficial. In a case-controlled study of 3033 patients with diabetes and cancer who were treated with anthracyclines, there was an incidence of cardiac events in 3% of patients taking SGLT-2 inhibitors compared to 20% incidence of cardiac events in the other patients, not taking SGLT-2 inhibitors [38]. Of course, these data are not conclusive. A prospective study would be needed to establish this relationship.

There are two approaches to limiting cardiotoxicity other than restricting the dose. One option is to monitor the patient for early signs of CTRCD [22] and then treat with medications with proven benefit for heart failure, commonly referred to as guideline-directed medical therapy (GDMT) [16, 39]. A second approach in persons thought to be at special risk would be to start the protective medication "up front" with the first dose of doxorubicin, continuing surveillance to avoid developing severe CTRCD. Treatment with the beta blockers and the ACE inhibitors or ARBs is often problematic as they can cause increased fatigue and relative hypotension, which seriously affects the quality of life. Even statins are associated with fatigue in some instances. The cardioprotective effect of these medications, at least with carvedilol, was greater if given within the first six months of cardiac dysfunction. Additionally, continuation of cardioprotective treatment is likely important. Withdrawal of carvedilol therapy after recovery of function, even after stopping the doxorubicin, was associated with deterioration of function that was not reliably reversed with resumption of the beta blocker [16]. GDMT drugs used to treat heart failure, may be difficult to use in patients with cancer as they may cause hypotension or fatigue, which are problematic in these patients. Often doses are limited or withheld unless there is a clear need for the protection.

A second, in many ways complementary approach to reducing the effect of doxorubicin on the heart, is to alter the administration of doxorubicin to limit cardiac toxicity while not depressing the effect on the tumor. One initial approach has been to modify the administration of doxorubicin to minimize high serum levels, which are thought to cause cardiac toxicity without improving tumor efficacy. Slow infusion [14, 40] that lowers peak serum levels of the doxorubicin has been used. Slow infusion is effective but expensive and requires more time in the hospital [14]. Liposomal formulations of doxorubicin have been developed to reduce the peak levels but have historically had limited availability and increased the cost of treatment.

Because the effects of doxorubicin on the cancer cells and the heart are thought to be different [41], it seemed reasonable that a drug could block the effects of doxorubicin on the heart without reducing its effect on tumors. Chelating agents, related to ethylene diamine tetra-acetic acid (EDTA), had been proposed as compounds which would possess antitumor activity [42]. Dexrazoxane, a bisdioxopiperazine derived from EDTA, was shown to be effective in pediatric cancer patients-achieving a complete remission in one patient with lymphocytic leukemia and cleared the blood of lymphoblasts in four [43].

In early clinical studies, dexrazoxane also appeared to ameliorate the cardiac toxicity of anthracyclines [44]. Several randomized studies, on relatively small numbers of patients, showed impressive cardiac protection without impairing tumor efficacy [45, 46]. It was subsequently accepted that dexrazoxane protected the heart from doxorubicin cardiotoxicity and likely did not decrease tumor efficacy, but because of the small size of the studies (130 randomized patients), the question of a possible reduction in tumor efficacy remained.

Two separate studies with the same protocol and same PI, in patients with breast cancer treated with fluorouracil, dexrazoxane and cyclophosphamide randomized to dexrazoxane or placebo were published in 1997, the response rate in one study was 46.8% in the dexrazoxane group compared to 60.5% in the placebo group, and in the second study was 57.3% vs. 49.3% [47]. There was no difference in "time to progression" or survival. During the study, after the cardioprotective effect was clear, a protocol amendment was introduced to allow patients randomized initially to placebo to be given dexrazoxane if additional doxorubicin was desired to continue to treat the cancer. With this change, giving dexrazoxane after a total of 300 mg/m2 of doxorubicin, patients receiving dexrazoxane had significantly less heart failure with higher doses of doxorubicin (3 vs. 22%) [48]. Based on this study, in 1995, dexrazoxane received approval for patients with breast cancer but only after 300 mg/M2 of doxorubicin had been administered.

There were genuine concerns with this more limited, dose-dependent approval, especially since it is known that cardiac damage can occur with the first infusion [49]. At a meeting of French and American oncologists and cardiologists in Paris in 2001 [50], the consensus opinion was that dexrazoxane was underutilized, in large part because of concern that dexrazoxane would decrease tumor efficacy. The participants further opined that the data did not support a decrease in tumor efficacy by dexrazoxane and they recommended that dexrazoxane be more widely utilized. It was recognized that the quality of the data even at that time was poor, reducing the confidence in these recommendations [51].

In the pediatric age group, dexrazoxane is begun at the onset of treatment in order to limit long-term cardiotoxicity because of the anticipated long-term survival in many patients and the anticipated high doses of doxorubicin required. For sarcomas in adults, doxorubicin remains the most effective treatment for advanced or metastatic sarcomas so that approaches to permit therapy by limiting cardiotoxicity are critical. A number of studies have evaluated "upfront" dexrazoxane, giving the dexrazoxane with the first dose of doxorubicin in sarcomas with no evidence for a reduction in efficacy. A preliminary analysis in a study of upfront dexrazoxane in patients with soft tissue sarcomas shows no decrease in progression-free survival in patients treated with upfront dexrazoxane [52] but more data are needed before this is established.

5. Mechanism of action of dexrazoxane

It has been believed that doxorubicin causes damage to the cardiac myocytes and the tumor through different mechanisms opening the possibility for a drug, which can protect the cardiac myocytes while not impairing the effectiveness of doxorubicin against the tumor. The initial construct suggested a major role in the production of free radicals by doxorubicin disrupting mitochondria and flooding the mitochondria with iron [53]. Dexrazoxane was introduced initially to chelate the iron and prevent this process. More recent studies show that doxorubicin manifests its tumorocidal actions and cardiotoxic actions primarily through interference with TOPII, an enzyme responsible for permitting the DNA to separate and come back together in mitosis [54]. There are two isomers: TOPIIα in the tumor and TOPIIβ in the heart and also in the tumor. Dexrazoxane, given before the doxorubicin, binds with the TOPIIβ so that the enzyme is not available to bind with the doxorubicin and the heart is protected. Dexrazoxane's cardioprotection appears to depend primarily on this mechanism, binding with TOPII rather than iron chelation. Martin et al. tested a drug similar to

DOI: http://dx.doi.org/10.5772/intechopen.1004240

dexrazoxane with its iron-binding properties but without interaction with TOPII. They found no cardioprotective effects of this drug in mice given doxorubicin [55]. Unfortunately, dexrazoxane also interacts to a lesser extent with TOPII2α in most tumors and may lower its levels in the tumors which would also reduce the target for doxorubicin [56]. However, the interaction of dexrazoxane with TOPIIα itself causes DNA damage response and DNA double-strand breaks, which are toxic to the tumor [57]. This interaction of dexrazoxane with the TOPIIα varies among tumor types so that one cannot predict with confidence that the tumor efficacy will be preserved uniformly across all cancers.

6. Administration of dexrazoxane

Dexrazoxane should be administered intravenously over 15 minutes rather than a one-time IV push [58]. The dosage ratio of dexrazoxane to doxorubicin is 10:1. It should be given 30 minutes to an hour before the doxorubicin. Dosing mechanisms are different in patients with renal and hepatic impairment. Typically, renal patients with estimated creatinine clearance lower than 40 mL/min have dexrazoxane dosages reduced by 50% [59]. The dosage ratio would also change to a 5:1 ratio. In terms of hepatic impairment, most notably in the setting of hyperbilirubinemia, dexrazoxane should also be dose reduced along with doxorubicin to maintain a 10:1 ratio. Dexrazoxane is only approved for use in patients with breast cancer who have gotten doses of doxorubicin of 300 mg/m^2 or more and continuing treatment with doxorubicin [7]. Of course, it is widely used in many types of cancer, especially soft tissue sarcomas where doxorubicin is the mainstay of therapy and strategy is to maximize the dose which can only be done safely if the heart is protected with dexrazoxane [14, 60]. Case reports in patients with severe cardiomyopathy prior to treatment and ongoing larger studies in patients with cancers other than breast are challenging the limitations of the original FDA approval [60, 61].

7. Adverse side effects of dexrazoxane

Dexrazoxane was originally developed as a chemotherapeutic agent, but was found to have serious toxicities at tumorocidal doses. Bone marrow suppression is one of the most common side effects. Much like with doxorubicin, leukopenia, neutropenia, granulocytopenia and thrombocytopenia may occur. The myelodysplastic syndrome has been reported. It can certainly be difficult to distinguish whether a side effect in a given patient is due to the dexrazoxane itself or doxorubicin, since both are given together [62]. However, aside from pain with injection, adverse effects are seen with about the same frequency as with doxorubicin alone [7]. Nonetheless, neutropenic fever (infection in the setting of decreased white blood cell count) has been reported in patients with dexrazoxane. Gastrointestinal distress such as nausea, vomiting and diarrhea have been described in patients taking the medication [63]. Injection site reactions such as pain, redness, swelling and irritation can also occur. Although rare, allergic reactions such as anaphylaxis, angioedema, skin reactions, bronchospasm, respiratory distress, hypotension and loss of consciousness have been reported [64]. Dexrazoxane might cause changes in liver function tests, indicating potential liver issues [65]. Some individuals may experience fatigue or weakness as a result of dexrazoxane treatment.

There have been concerns that dexrazoxane might increase the risk of secondary malignancies, especially in pediatric populations. More specifically, acute myeloid leukemia (AML) and myelodysplastic syndrome (MDS) have been reported in patients given dexrazoxane. A randomized clinical trial by Tebbi et al. suggested that pediatric Hodgkin's lymphoma patients have an increased risk of secondary malignancies stated above when treated with dexrazoxane [66]. However, Lipshultz et al. criticized this trial due to having weak statistical power [67] and the question remains in doubt. Dexrazoxane can cause damage to the fetus and in studies with pregnant rabbits and mice effects on the fetus and maternal toxicity were seen at lower doses than the clinically recommended dose. Dexrazoxane can be given to pregnant women but patients need to be appraised of the risk to the fetus. Infertility in males is also a concern with dexrazoxane [58, 68].

8. Extravasation injury of anthracyclines: treatment with dexrazoxane

Extravasation of doxorubicin causes necrosis of the tissue involved, which untreated may need surgical repair. The mechanism of this is not clear but may be related to damage to DNA binding mechanisms leading to local inflammation and tissue necrosis [69]. This damage is very similar histologically to the damage of ionizing radiation. Dexrazoxane intravenously, not locally, has been shown to limit this problem [70, 71]. The mechanism of how dexrazoxane promotes recovery from extravasation is not clear. Mice models have suggested that the interaction between dexrazoxane and TOPII is not important in protecting from anthracycline extravasation local injury/necrosis [72]. It is more likely that the iron-chelation or direct antioxidant effect likely plays a role in protection against extravasation. Thirty-six patients with anthracycline extravasation were given dexrazoxane intravenously in two clinical trials. These patients were then given multiple infusions of dexrazoxane with appropriate healing and recovery. Only one patient required surgical debridement in the treatment arm [73]. Because of these studies, the FDA quickly approved dexrazoxane to treat anthracycline extravasation.

9. Summary/conclusion

Doxorubicin remains a very important drug in the cancer armamentarium, especially for soft tissue sarcomas, where it is the most important agent, but also in breast, lymphomas and pediatric cancers. In tumors responsive to doxorubicin, the main limitation to treatment is severe and progressive cardiac dysfunction. Thus, it is essential to protect against cardiac toxicity to permit effective dosing of the doxorubicin. While there are a number of therapeutic approaches to mitigating cardiac damage, namely medications used for GDMT for heart failure, as well as statins and possibly SGLT-2 inhibitors, the most effective approach is with dexrazoxane, which protects the heart without seriously impairing tumor efficacy. While more research is needed to better understand both the mechanism of doxorubicin's tumorocidal effects as well as the mechanism of its cardiac toxicity, at present dexrazoxane given with doxorubicin appears to protect the heart without affecting tumor efficacy.

Author details

Ronald J. Krone[1*], Azim Merchant[2] and Joshua D. Mitchell[1]

1 School of Medicine, Washington University, St. Louis, Missouri, USA

2 School of Medicine, Barnes-Jewish Hospital, Washington University, St. Louis, Missouri, USA

*Address all correspondence to: rkrone@wustl.edu

References

[1] Tan C, Etcubanas E, Wollner N, Rosen G, Gilladoga A, Showel J, et al. Adriamycin – An antitumor antibiotic in the treatment of neoplastic diseases. Cancer. 1973;**32**(1):9-17

[2] Sritharan S, Sivalingam N. A comprehensive review on time-tested anticancer drug doxorubicin. Life Sciences. 2021;**278**:119527

[3] Benjamin RS, Wiernik PH, Bachur NR. Adriamycin: A new effective agent in the therapy of disseminated sarcomas. Medical and Pediatric Oncology. 1975;**1**(1):63-76

[4] Chen GL, Yang L, Rowe TC, Halligan BD, Tewey KM, Liu LF. Nonintercalative antitumor drugs interfere with the breakage-Reunion reaction of mammalian DNA topoisomerase II. The Journal of Biological Chemistry. 1984;**259**(21):13560-13566

[5] Tewey KM, Rowe TC, Yang L, Halligan BD, Liu LF. Adriamycin-induced DNA damage mediated by mammalian DNA topoisomerase II. Science. 1984;**226**(4673):466-468

[6] Kciuk M, Gielecinska A, Mujwar S, Kolat D, Kaluzinska-Kolat Z, Celik I, et al. Doxorubicin-an agent with multiple mechanisms of anticancer activity. Cells. 2023;**12**(4):259-289

[7] Pfizer. Zinecard (dexrazoxane) for injection. In: Highlights of Prescribing Information. New York, NY: Pfizer, Inc.; 2014. pp. 1-13. Available from: https://www.accessdata.fda.gov/drugsatfda_docs/label/2014/020212s017lbl.pdf

[8] Asensio-Lopez MC, Soler F, Pascual-Figal D, Fernandez-Belda F, Lax A. Doxorubicin-induced oxidative stress: The protective effect of nicorandil on HL-1 cardiomyocytes. PLoS One. 2017;**12**(2):e0172803

[9] Murabito A, Hirsch E, Ghigo A. Mechanisms of anthracycline-induced cardiotoxicity: Is mitochondrial dysfunction the answer? Frontiers in Cardiovascular Medicine. 2020;**7**:35

[10] Gewirtz DA. A critical evaluation of the mechanisms of action proposed for the antitumor effects of the anthracycline antibiotics adriamycin and daunorubicin. Biochemical Pharmacology. 1999;**57**(7):727-741

[11] Solem LE, Henry TR, Wallace KB. Disruption of mitochondrial calcium homeostasis following chronic doxorubicin administration. Toxicology and Applied Pharmacology. 1994;**129**(2):214-222

[12] Von Hoff DD, Layard MW, Basa P, Davis HL Jr, Von Hoff AL, Rozencweig M, et al. Risk factors for doxorubicin-induced congestive heart failure. Annals of Internal Medicine. 1979;**91**(5):710-717

[13] Schwartz RG, McKenzie WB, Alexander J, Sager P, D'Souza A, Manatunga A, et al. Congestive heart failure and left ventricular dysfunction complicating doxorubicin therapy. Seven-year experience using serial radionuclide angiocardiography. The American Journal of Medicine. 1987;**82**(6):1109-1118

[14] Benjamin RS, Minotti G. Doxorubicin-dexrazoxane from day 1 for soft-tissue sarcomas: The road to Cardioprotection. Clinical Cancer Research. 2021;**27**(14):3809-3811

[15] Lyon AR, Lopez-Fernandez T, Couch LS, Asteggiano R, Aznar MC,

Bergler-Klein J, et al. 2022 ESC guidelines on cardio-oncology developed in collaboration with the European Hematology Association (EHA), the European Society for Therapeutic Radiology and Oncology (ESTRO) and the international cardio-oncology society (IC-OS). European Heart Journal. 2022;**43**(41):4229-4361

[16] Cardinale D, Colombo A, Lamantia G, Colombo N, Civelli M, De Giacomi G, et al. Anthracycline-induced cardiomyopathy clinical relevance and response to pharmacologic therapy. Journal of the American College of Cardiology. 2010;**55**(3):213-220

[17] Curigliano G, Lenihan D, Fradley M, Ganatra S, Barac A, Blaes A, et al. Management of cardiac disease in cancer patients throughout oncological treatment: ESMO consensus recommendations. Annals of Oncology. 2020;**31**(2):171-190

[18] Baldassarre LA, Ganatra S, Lopez-Mattei J, Yang EH, Zaha VG, Wong TC, et al. Advances in multimodality imaging in cardio-oncology. Journal of the American College of Cardiology. 2022;**80**(16):1560-1578

[19] Plana JC, Galderisi M, Barac A, Ewer MS, Ky B, Scherrer-Crosbie M, et al. Expert consensus for multimodality imaging evaluation of adult patients during and after cancer therapy: A report from the American Society of Echocardiography and the European Association of Cardiovascular Imaging. Journal of the American Society of Echocardiography. 2014;**27**(9):911-939

[20] Thavendiranathan P, Grant AD, Negishi T, Plana JC, Popovic ZB, Marwick TH. Reproducibility of echocardiographic techniques for sequential assessment of left ventricular ejection fraction and volumes: Application to patients undergoing cancer chemotherapy. Journal of the American College of Cardiology. 2013;**61**(1):77-84

[21] Liu JE, Barac A, Thavendiranathan P, Scherrer-Crosbie M. Strain imaging in cardio-oncology. JACC CardioOncology. 2020;**2**(5):677-689

[22] Herrmann J, Lenihan D, Armenian S, Barac A, Blaes A, Cardinale D, et al. Defining cardiovascular toxicities of cancer therapies: An international cardio-oncology society (IC-OS) consensus statement. European Heart Journal. 2022;**43**(4):280-299

[23] Lefrak EA, Pitha J, Rosenheim S, Gottlieb JA. A clinicopathologic analysis of adriamycin cardiotoxicity. Cancer. 1973;**32**(2):302-314

[24] Hamo CE, Bloom MW, Cardinale D, Ky B, Nohria A, Baer L, et al. Cancer therapy-related cardiac dysfunction and heart failure: Part 2: Prevention, treatment, guidelines, and future directions. Circulation. Heart Failure. 2016;**9**(2):e002843

[25] Krone RJ. Protecting the heart in Cancer patients: The role of cardio-oncology. European Medical Journal Cardiology. 2017;**5**(1):47-52

[26] Curigliano G, Cardinale D, Dent S, Criscitiello C, Aseyev O, Lenihan D, et al. Cardiotoxicity of anticancer treatments: Epidemiology, detection, and management. CA: a Cancer Journal for Clinicians. 2016;**66**(4):309-325

[27] Kalam K, Marwick TH. Role of cardioprotective therapy for prevention of cardiotoxicity with chemotherapy: A systematic review and meta-analysis. European Journal of Cancer. 2013;**49**(13):2900-2909

[28] Bosch X, Rovira M, Sitges M, Domenech A, Ortiz-Perez JT, de

Caralt TM, et al. Enalapril and carvedilol for preventing chemotherapy-induced left ventricular systolic dysfunction in patients with malignant hemopathies: The OVERCOME trial (preventiOn of left ventricular dysfunction with enalapril and caRvedilol in patients submitted to intensive ChemOtherapy for the treatment of malignant hEmopathies). Journal of the American College of Cardiology. 2013;**61**(23):2355-2362

[29] Kaya MG, Ozkan M, Gunebakmaz O, Akkaya H, Kaya EG, Akpek M, et al. Protective effects of nebivolol against anthracycline-induced cardiomyopathy: A randomized control study. International Journal of Cardiology. 2013;**167**(5):2306-2310

[30] Gulati G, Heck SL, Ree AH, Hoffmann P, Schulz-Menger J, Fagerland MW, et al. Prevention of cardiac dysfunction during adjuvant breast cancer therapy (PRADA): A 2 x 2 factorial, randomized, placebo-controlled, double-blind clinical trial of candesartan and metoprolol. European Heart Journal. 2016;**37**(21):1671-1680

[31] Georgakopoulos P, Roussou P, Matsakas E, Karavidas A, Anagnostopoulos N, Marinakis T, et al. Cardioprotective effect of metoprolol and enalapril in doxorubicin-treated lymphoma patients: A prospective, parallel-group, randomized, controlled study with 36-month follow-up. American Journal of Hematology. 2010;**85**(11):894-896

[32] Cardinale D, Colombo A, Sandri MT, Lamantia G, Colombo N, Civelli M, et al. Prevention of high-dose chemotherapy-induced cardiotoxicity in high-risk patients by angiotensin-converting enzyme inhibition. Circulation. 2006;**114**(23):2474-2481

[33] Nakamae H, Tsumura K, Terada Y, Nakane T, Nakamae M, Ohta K, et al. Notable effects of angiotensin II receptor blocker, valsartan, on acute cardiotoxic changes after standard chemotherapy with cyclophosphamide, doxorubicin, vincristine, and prednisolone. Cancer. 2005;**104**(11):2492-2498

[34] Cadeddu C, Piras A, Mantovani G, Deidda M, Dessi M, Madeddu C, et al. Protective effects of the angiotensin II receptor blocker telmisartan on epirubicin-induced inflammation, oxidative stress, and early ventricular impairment. American Heart Journal. 2010;**160**(3):e481-e487

[35] Akpek M, Ozdogru I, Sahin O, Inanc M, Dogan A, Yazici C, et al. Protective effects of spironolactone against anthracycline-induced cardiomyopathy. European Journal of Heart Failure. 2015;**17**(1):81-89

[36] Obasi M, Abovich A, Vo JB, Gao Y, Papatheodorou SI, Nohria A, et al. Statins to mitigate cardiotoxicity in cancer patients treated with anthracyclines and/or trastuzumab: A systematic review and meta-analysis. Cancer Causes & Control: CCC. 2021;**32**(12):1395-1405

[37] Obasi M, Abovich A, Vo JB, Gao Y, Papatheodorou SI, Nohria A, et al. Correction to: Statins to mitigate cardiotoxicity in cancer patients treated with anthracyclines and/or trastuzumab: A systematic review and meta-analysis. Cancer Causes & Control: CCC. 2021;**32**(12):1407-1409

[38] Gongora CA, Drobni ZD, Quinaglia Araujo Costa Silva T, Zafar A, Gong J, Zlotoff DA, et al. Sodium-glucose Co-Transporter-2 inhibitors and cardiac outcomes among patients treated with anthracyclines. JACC: Heart Failure. 2022;**10**(8):559-567

[39] Heidenreich PA, Bozkurt B, Aguilar D, Allen LA, Byun JJ,

Colvin MM, et al. 2022 AHA/ACC/HFSA guideline for the Management of Heart Failure: A report of the American College of Cardiology/American Heart Association joint committee on clinical practice guidelines. Journal of the American College of Cardiology. 2022;**79**(17):e263-e421

[40] Zalupski M, Metch B, Balcerzak S, Fletcher WS, Chapman R, Bonnet JD, et al. Phase III comparison of doxorubicin and dacarbazine given by bolus versus infusion in patients with soft-tissue sarcomas: A southwest oncology group study. Journal of the National Cancer Institute. 1991;**83**(13):926-932

[41] Hellmann K. Anthracycline cardiotoxicity prevention by dexrazoxane: Breakthrough of a barrier--sharpens antitumor profile and therapeutic index. Journal of Clinical Oncology. 1996;**14**(2):332-333

[42] Creighton AM, Hellmann K, Whitecross S. Antitumour activity in a series of bisdiketopiperazines. Nature. 1969;**222**(5191):384-385

[43] Holcenberg JS, Tutsch KD, Earhart RH, Ungerleider RS, Kamen BA, Pratt CB, et al. Phase I study of ICRF-187 in pediatric cancer patients and comparison of its pharmacokinetics in children and adults. Cancer Treatment Reports. 1986;**70**(6):703-709

[44] Poster DS, Penta JS, Bruno S, Macdonald JS. ICRF-187 in clinical oncology. Cancer Clinical Trials. 1981;**4**(2):143-146

[45] Wexler LH, Andrich MP, Venzon D, Berg SL, Weaver-McClure L, Chen CC, et al. Randomized trial of the cardioprotective agent ICRF-187 in pediatric sarcoma patients treated with doxorubicin. Journal of Clinical Oncology. 1996;**14**(2):362-372

[46] Speyer JL, Green MD, Kramer E, Rey M, Sanger J, Ward C, et al. Protective effect of the bispiperazinedione ICRF-187 against doxorubicin-induced cardiac toxicity in women with advanced breast cancer. The New England Journal of Medicine. 1988;**319**(12):745-752

[47] Swain SM, Whaley FS, Gerber MC, Weisberg S, York M, Spicer D, et al. Cardioprotection with dexrazoxane for doxorubicin-containing therapy in advanced breast cancer. Journal of Clinical Oncology. 1997;**15**(4):1318-1332

[48] Swain SM, Whaley FS, Gerber MC, Ewer MS, Bianchine JR, Gams RA. Delayed administration of dexrazoxane provides cardioprotection for patients with advanced breast cancer treated with doxorubicin-containing therapy. Journal of Clinical Oncology. 1997;**15**(4):1333-1340

[49] Unverferth BJ, Magorien RD, Balcerzak SP, Leier CV, Unverferth DV. Early changes in human myocardial nuclei after doxorubicin. Cancer. 1983;**52**(2):215-221

[50] Swain SM, Vici P. The current and future role of dexrazoxane as a cardioprotectant in anthracycline treatment: Expert panel review. Journal of Cancer Research and Clinical Oncology. 2004;**130**(1):1-7

[51] Macedo AVS, Hajjar LA, Lyon AR, Nascimento BR, Putzu A, Rossi L, Costa RB, Landoni G, Nogueira-Rodrigues A, Ribeiro ALP. Efficacy of dexrazoxane in preventing anthracycline cardiotoxicity in breast Cancer. JACC: CardioOncology. 2019;**1**(1):68-79

[52] Van Tine BA, Hirbe AC, Oppelt P, Frith AE, Rathore R, Mitchell JD, et al. Interim analysis of the phase II study: Noninferiority study of doxorubicin with

upfront dexrazoxane plus Olaratumab for advanced or metastatic soft-tissue sarcoma. Clinical Cancer Research. 2021;**27**(14):3854-3860

[53] Sawyer DB, Peng X, Chen B, Pentassuglia L, Lim CC. Mechanisms of anthracycline cardiac injury: Can we identify strategies for cardioprotection? Progress in Cardiovascular Diseases. 2010;**53**(2):105-113

[54] Sawyer DB. Anthracyclines and heart failure. The New England Journal of Medicine. 2013;**368**(12):1154-1156

[55] Martin E, Thougaard AV, Grauslund M, Jensen PB, Bjorkling F, Hasinoff BB, et al. Evaluation of the topoisomerase II-inactive bisdioxopiperazine ICRF-161 as a protectant against doxorubicin-induced cardiomyopathy. Toxicology. 2009;**255**(1-2):72-79

[56] Deng S, Yan T, Jendrny C, Nemecek A, Vincetic M, Godtel-Armbrust U, et al. Dexrazoxane may prevent doxorubicin-induced DNA damage via depleting both topoisomerase II isoforms. BMC Cancer. 2014;**14**:842

[57] Deng S, Yan T, Nikolova T, Fuhrmann D, Nemecek A, Godtel-Armbrust U, et al. The catalytic topoisomerase II inhibitor dexrazoxane induces DNA breaks, ATF3 and the DNA damage response in cancer cells. British Journal of Pharmacology. 2015;**172**(9):2246-2257

[58] Eneh C, Lekkala MR. Dexrazoxane. In: *StatPearls (Internet) Treasure Island*. StatPearls: FL; 2023

[59] Brier ME, Gaylor SK, McGovren JP, Glue P, Fang A, Aronoff GR. Pharmacokinetics of dexrazoxane in subjects with impaired kidney function. Journal of Clinical Pharmacology. 2011;**51**(5):731-738

[60] Jones RL, Wagner AJ, Kawai A, Tamura K, Shahir A, Van Tine BA, et al. Prospective evaluation of doxorubicin cardiotoxicity in patients with advanced soft-tissue sarcoma treated in the ANNOUNCE phase III randomized trial. Clinical Cancer Research. 2021;**27**(14):3861-3866

[61] Banerjee R, Lo M, Klein L, Aras M, Logan AC. Anthracyclines in a patient with acute leukemia and severe cardiomyopathy requiring mechanical support: A case report. Journal of Oncology Pharmacy Practice. 2022;**28**(3):729-732

[62] Spalato Ceruso M, Napolitano A, Silletta M, Mazzocca A, Valeri S, Improta L, et al. Use of cardioprotective dexrazoxane is associated with increased myelotoxicity in anthracycline-treated soft-tissue sarcoma patients. Chemotherapy. 2019;**64**(2):105-109

[63] Curran CF, Narang PK, Reynolds RD. Toxicity profile of dexrazoxane (Zinecard, ICRF-187, ADR-529, NSC-169780), a modulator of doxorubicin cardiotoxicity. Cancer Treatment Reviews. 1991;**18**(4):241-252

[64] Leoni V, Santini D, Vincenzi B, Grilli C, Onori N, Tonini G. Anaphylaxis to dexrazoxane (ICRF-187) following three previous uncomplicated infusions. Allergy. 2004;**59**(2):241

[65] Zima T, Tesar V, Sherwood R, Sood A, Au LC, Richardson PJ, et al. Acute dosage with dexrazoxane, but not doxorubicin, is associated with increased rates of hepatic protein synthesis in vivo. Toxicologic Pathology. 2001;**29**(6):591-599

[66] Tebbi CK, London WB, Friedman D, Villaluna D, De Alarcon PA, Constine LS, et al. Dexrazoxane-associated risk for acute myeloid leukemia/myelodysplastic syndrome and other secondary malignancies in pediatric Hodgkin's

disease. Journal of Clinical Oncology. 2007;**25**(5):493-500

[67] Lipshultz SE, Lipsitz SR, Orav EJ. Dexrazoxane-associated risk for secondary malignancies in pediatric Hodgkin's disease: A claim without compelling evidence. Journal of Clinical Oncology. 2007;**25**(21):3179

[68] Levi M, Tzabari M, Savion N, Stemmer SM, Shalgi R, Ben-Aharon I. Dexrazoxane exacerbates doxorubicin-induced testicular toxicity. Reproduction. 2015;**150**(4):357-366

[69] Kreidieh FY, Moukadem HA, El Saghir NS. Overview, prevention and management of chemotherapy extravasation. World Journal of Clinical Oncology. 2016;**7**(1):87-97

[70] Kane RC, McGuinn WD Jr, Dagher R, Justice R, Pazdur R. Dexrazoxane (Totect): FDA review and approval for the treatment of accidental extravasation following intravenous anthracycline chemotherapy. The Oncologist. 2008;**13**(4):445-450

[71] Jordan K, Behlendorf T, Mueller F, Schmoll HJ. Anthracycline extravasation injuries: Management with dexrazoxane. Therapeutics and Clinical Risk Management. 2009;**5**(2):361-366

[72] Langer SW, Jensen PB, Sehested M. Other uses of dexrazoxane: Savene, the first proven antidote against anthracycline extravasation injuries. Cardiovascular Toxicology. 2007;**7**(2):151-153

[73] Mouridsen HT, Langer SW, Buter J, Eidtmann H, Rosti G, de Wit M, et al. Treatment of anthracycline extravasation with Savene (dexrazoxane): Results from two prospective clinical multicentre studies. Annals of Oncology. 2007;**18**(3):546-550

Section 2

Drug Delivery Technologies

Chapter 7

Fundamentals Applications of Controlled Release Drug Delivery

Muhammad Saeed Jan, Waqas Alam and Madeeha Shabnam

Abstract

The advancement of pharmacology and pharmacokinetics highlighted the important role of drug release kinetics in the determination of therapeutic outcomes of treatments. The advent of modified release dosage forms marked a significant innovation. Technological progressions in coating methods gained momentum in the late 1800s, encompassing innovations like sugar and enteric coatings applied to pills and tablets. Subsequent advancements led to the refinement of enteric coatings for tablets, which eventually evolved into the incorporation of a secondary drug within the sugar coating layer. However, the initial patent for oral-sustained release formulations was awarded to Lipowski. His formulation comprised miniature-coated beads designed to achieve gradual and consistent drug release. This concept was subsequently refined by Blythe, leading to the introduction of the first commercially available sustained release product. Over the last three decades, the escalating complexities associated with bringing new drugs to market, coupled with the recognized merits of Controlled Release Drug Delivery Systems (CRDDS). Presently, oral controlled drug delivery systems have emerged as significant avenues, particularly for compounds characterized by high water solubility and abbreviated biological half-lives. Beyond oral administration, diverse routes such as transdermal, ocular, vaginal, and parenteral approaches are utilized for controlled release of various therapeutic agents.

Keywords: dose-activity relationship, sustained drug concentration, control drug delivery, drug release rate, transdermal drug delivery

1. Introduction

Controlled drug delivery systems offer various advantages such as regulating drug concentrations effectively, reducing the frequency of administrations, maximizing drug utilization, and enhancing patient adherence [1]. Besides that, these systems also display potential drawbacks including material toxicity or lack of biocompatibility, generation of undesirable degradation by-products, necessity for surgical procedures for system implantation or removal, likelihood of patient discomfort due to the delivery device [2], and the elevated cost associated with controlled-release systems relative to conventional pharmaceutical formulations [3]. The optimal drug delivery system should possess qualities of inertness, biocompatibility, mechanical robustness, patient comfort, high drug loading capacity, prevention of unintended release, ease of administration and removal, and simplicity in fabrication and sterilization [4]. The primary objective of early controlled-release systems was to establish a drug delivery profile that would sustain elevated drug concentrations in the bloodstream across an extended duration. In conventional drug delivery approaches, blood drug levels exhibit a pattern characterized by post-administration escalation followed by a subsequent decline until the subsequent dose is administered. A fundamental principle of traditional drug administration is to maintain the blood concentration of the drug within a range bounded by an upper threshold, which could signify a toxic concentration, and a lower threshold below which the drug's efficacy diminishes [5].

2. Terminology or definition of control release dosage forms

According to the USP, modified-release (MR) dosage form is a formulation selected to achieve therapeutic or practical goals that surpass the capabilities of conventional dosage forms like solutions, ointments, or rapidly dissolving formulations, based on its tailored drug release attributes concerning temporal progression and/or spatial localization [6]. A category within the domain of modified-release (MR) dosage forms is represented by the extended-release (ER) dosage form [6]. This category is characterized by the capability to achieve a minimum reduction of twice in dosing frequency or substantial enhancements in patient adherence and therapeutic efficacy, in contrast to conventional dosage forms such as solutions or rapid drug-releasing formulations [7]. The nomenclature "controlled release (CR)," "prolonged release," "sustained or slow release (SR)," and "long-acting (LA)" have been interchangeably employed to denote the concept of "extended release." Controlled drug delivery pertains to a mechanism by which a specific drug is administered either locally or systemically at a predetermined and regulated rate over a defined duration [8].

A prolonged-release pharmaceutical formulation administers a therapeutic dose of a medication across an elongated time period [9].

Prolonged release or sustained release systems, designed solely to extend therapeutic drug concentrations within blood or tissues over an extended interval, do not fall under the categorization of controlled-release systems as per this delineation. They are discernible from rate-controlled drug delivery systems, which possess the capacity to accurately determine *in vivo* release rates and durations through straightforward *in vitro* assessments [10].

Controlled drug delivery pertains to the regulated administration of a drug at a predetermined rate over a specified timeframe. Controlled release exhibits a zero-order release profile, signifying consistent drug release over time regardless of concentration fluctuations. Sustained release dosage forms, on the other hand, encompass a specific drug delivery configuration where an initial drug dose is promptly released to achieve a rapid therapeutic response. Subsequently, a gradual release of the remaining maintenance dose ensues, ensuring a prolonged but non-constant therapeutic concentration. Sustained release conveys the gradual dispensation of a drug throughout a designated temporal interval. This characteristic may or may not entail controlled-release attributes [11].

In contrast, drug targeting can be conceptualized as a variant of controlled release due to its capacity to exert localized control over drug release within the physiological context [12].

3. Rationale

The fundamental principle behind a controlled-release drug delivery system is to enhance the drug's biopharmaceutical, pharmacokinetic, and pharmacodynamics attributes to optimize its efficacy. This optimization aims to minimize adverse effects while achieving disease management or cure in the swiftest feasible duration, utilizing the smallest feasible drug quantity, and selecting the most appropriate administration route. Immediate release drug delivery systems exhibit certain limitations, including the absence of dose maintenance, lack of controlled-release kinetics, and inability to precisely target specific sites within the body [13]. An ideal drug delivery system should ensure the drug's dispensation aligns with the body's requirements throughout a designated treatment period. This entails delivering the drug at a rate that corresponds to the body's needs while considering the specific duration of therapy [14].

4. Advantages of controlled-release dosage forms

4.1 Clinical advantages

- Reduces the frequency of drug administration
- Improvement in the compliance of a patient
- Minimizing fluctuation of drug level in the blood
- Decreasing drug utilization as compared with conventional therapy
- Diminished drug accumulation during chronic treatment
- Decrease in the toxicity of the drug whether local or systemic
- Stabilized patient's medical condition due to the achievement of uniform drug levels
- Enhanced bioavailability for specific drugs due to spatial regulation
- Cost-effectiveness for both healthcare provider and the patient (**Figures 1** and **2**)

4.2 Commercial/industrial advantages

- Demonstration of innovative and technological forefront
- Extension of product life cycle
- Establishment of product distinctiveness
- Broadening of market reach
- Extension of Patent protection

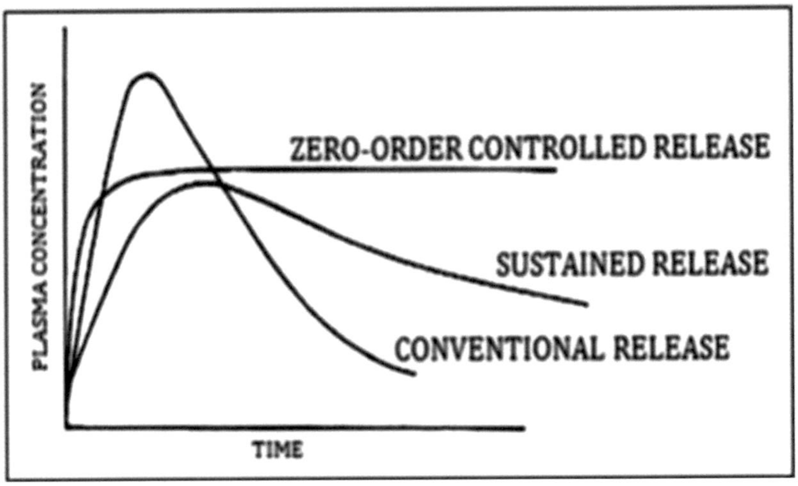

Figure 1.
Plasma drug concentration-time profile [15].

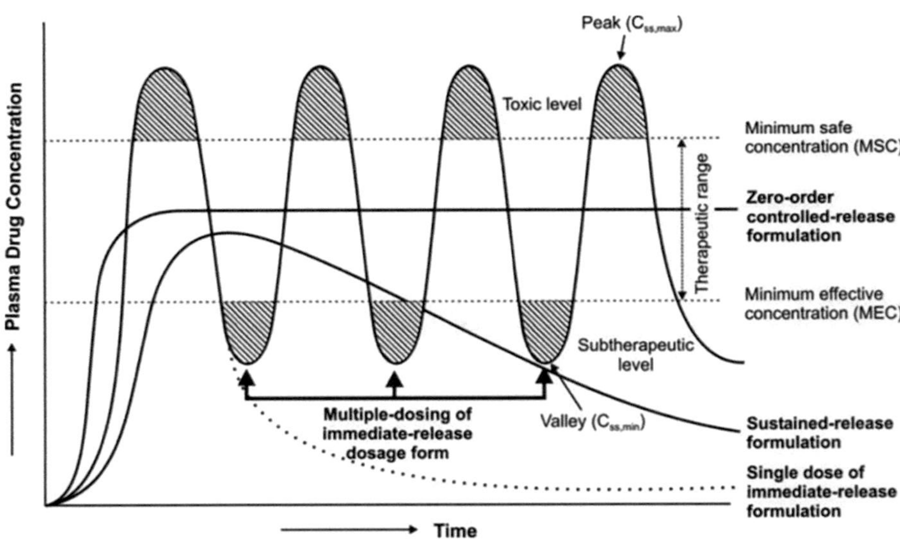

Figure 2.
A hypothetical plasma concentration-time profile from conventional multiple dosing and an ideal controlled delivery formulation [16].

4.3 Disadvantages of CRDDS

- Delayed initiation of drug effects
- Potential risk of dose release surge with inadequate formulation strategy
- Elevated susceptibility to first-pass metabolism

- Augmented reliance on gastrointestinal residence duration of dosage form
- Possible challenge in precise dose adaptation in certain scenarios
- Elevated cost per individual dose compared to conventional formulations
- Not all drugs are amenable to extended-release formulation
- Drug selection of drug for the preparation of extended-release dosage form is the crucial step. Drugs having following characteristics are not suitable for extended-release formulations.

5. Designing controlled release per oral drug delivery systems: Biopharmaceutic and pharmacokinetic aspects

Controlled-release oral medication delivery systems are of paramount importance in enhancing the therapeutic effectiveness and ensuring patient adherence to pharmaceutical goods. The design of these systems must take into account important factors related to biopharmaceutics and pharmacokinetics, as these factors govern the processes of drug absorption, distribution, metabolism, and elimination in the human body [17].

5.1 Biological half-life (t ½)

The biological half-life, commonly known as the "half-life," is a pharmacokinetic variable that characterizes the duration required for the concentration of a medicine or chemical within the organism to diminish by 50%. The topic being discussed holds significant importance in the fields of pharmacology and medicine, as it plays a pivotal role in determining the duration of a drug's activity within the body and the frequency at which it needs be provided to sustain therapeutic levels. The shorter the half-life (t ½) of a drug, the greater the variations observed between the highest steady-state concentration and the minimum steady-state concentration upon repeated administration. Therefore, it is necessary to increase the frequency of administration of the medication product [18].

5.2 Minimum effective concentration (MEC)

The term "minimum effective concentration" (MEC) pertains to the lowest concentration of a chemical or treatment within the human body that is necessary to elicit a therapeutic response. Stated differently, the minimal concentration of a pharmaceutical substance that elicits the intended therapeutic effect is referred to as the minimum effective concentration. This notion holds significant importance within the fields of pharmacology and medicine, as it aids healthcare practitioners in ascertaining the suitable dosage and administration regimen for a certain prescription [19].

Beyond the minimum effective concentration (MEC), the medicine may fail to manifest its intended therapeutic efficacy, resulting in insufficient treatment.

Conversely, concentrations over the minimum effective concentration (MEC) may lead to an elevated likelihood of unfavorable consequences, without necessarily yielding any supplementary therapeutic advantages. The objective is to sustain the concentration of the medicine within a therapeutic range, wherein the advantages surpass the potential drawbacks [20].

5.3 Dose size and extent of duration

As the period of treatment increases, there is a corresponding need for an increased total dose per unit delivery method. Therefore, there exists a constraint on the quantity of medication that may feasibly be included into such a system [21].

5.4 Relatively long $t_{1/2}$ or fluctuation desired at steady state

There exists a perspective among certain individuals that medications with a half-life of 12 h or longer do not require or provide any utility for either a sustained release (SR) or a controlled-release drug delivery system (CRDDS). This assertion is unfounded as there exist two scenarios in which a 12 or 24 CRDDS appears to be warranted:

1. A pharmaceutical compound with a half-life ranging from 12 to 72 h could potentially be developed for a controlled-release drug delivery system (CRDDS) that allows for administration every two to three days. The rate at which the blood level time curve decreases following the elimination of the medication from the body is contingent upon the drug's half-life (t ½). The natural variation between the maximum and minimum concentrations of Css can result in a rather significant impact, specifically by introducing a slow-release mechanism that prolongs the elimination process [22].

2. Certain drugs having a half-life (t1/2) ranging from 20 to 100 h, which are intended for extended administration, exhibit a preference for minimizing fluctuations between peak and trough concentrations under steady-state circumstances. States may prescribe medications either with the intention of attaining a specific treatment outcome or due to the limited breadth of the therapeutic range [23].

6. Required biopharmaceutical characteristics of the drug to meet CDDS criteria

6.1 Molecular weight

Convective transport enables the passage of small molecules across membrane holes. This phenomenon is relevant to both the liberation of drugs from the pharmaceutical formulation and their passage across a biological membrane. In the context of biological membranes, it has been observed that spherical molecules are often limited to a molecular weight of 150, whereas chain-like compounds are limited to a molecular weight of 400 [24].

6.2 Solubility

In order for absorption mechanisms to occur, it is important that the drug is available in a solute form at the specific site of absorption. In the preformulation study, it is imperative to ascertain the drug's solubility across different pH levels. When the solubility of a substance is below 0.1 μg/ml in an acidic media, it is anticipated that there will be inconsistent and diminished bioavailability. When the solubility of a substance is below 0.01 μg/ml, it is probable that absorption and availability are mostly governed by limitations in dissolving [25]. Therefore, the underlying factor driving dissemination may be insufficient. Passive diffusion from the small intestine appears to facilitate effective absorption of medicines following oral administration, provided that the non-ionized form constitutes a minimum of 0.1 to 1% of the medication.

6.3 Apparent partition coefficient (APC)

In order for drugs to be absorbed through passive diffusion, it is necessary for them to possess a minimum apparent partition coefficient (APC). There exists a positive correlation between the apparent partition coefficient (APC) in an n-octanol/buffer system and the rate of drug flux over a membrane. The determination of the acid dissociation constant (APC) is necessary across the whole pH spectrum within the gastrointestinal (GI) tract. The application of the apparent partition coefficient (APC) is necessary for the evaluation of drug distribution between controlled-release drug delivery systems (CRDDS) and the biological fluid [26].

6.4 Absorption mechanism

In order for a drug to be considered a viable candidate for per oral controlled-release drug delivery systems (CRDDS), it is imperative that its absorption process occurs *via* diffusion across the entirety of the gastrointestinal (GI) tract. The term "diffusion" in this context pertains to the process of absorption, which occurs through two distinct pathways: partitioning into the lipid membrane (transcellular) or travelling through water-filled channels (paracellular). The occurrence of absorption from all segments of the gastrointestinal (GI) tract is of significant importance, and this process can be influenced by various factors such as the drug's pKa, the pH level in the specific segment, the binding of the drug to mucus, and the rate of blood flow. The absorption process exhibits a strong reliance on the hydrodynamics within the gastrointestinal lumen [27].

6.5 Pharmacokinetic and elimination half life (t ½)

Pharmaceutical substances characterized by a half-life of 8 h are considered highly compatible with controlled-release drug delivery systems (CRDDS). If the half-life (t ½) is shorter than 1 h, it is possible that the required dose size for a dosage form intended to last for 12 or 24 h may be excessively large. If the half-life (t ½) of a substance is significantly lengthy, the use of controlled-release drug delivery systems (CRDDS) is generally unnecessary, unless the purpose is just to minimize fluctuations in steady-state blood concentrations [28].

6.6 Total clearance (CL)

Clearance (CL) is a pharmacokinetic parameter that quantifies the rate at which a drug is eliminated from the body by measuring the volume of distribution that is cleared of the drug over a specific period of time. The important parameter for evaluating the necessary dose rate for continuous release drug delivery systems and predicting the concentration in a steady state is the subject of discussion [29].

6.7 Terminal disposition rate constant (Ke or λz)

The terminal disposition rate constant, also known as the elimination rate constant, can be derived from the half-life (t ½) and is necessary for the prediction of a time-dependent blood level pattern [30].

6.8 Apparent volume of distribution (Vz)

The Vz is the theoretical volume that a pharmaceutical substance would occupy if it were dissolved at an equivalent concentration to that observed in the bloodstream. The proportionality constant that establishes the relationship between the quantity of a drug present in the body and the observed concentration in the bloodstream. Within the trio of CL, Vz, and t ½, it can be observed that the former two parameters function as independent variables, while the latter parameter serves as the dependent variable [31].

In order to forecast the concentration time profile, it is necessary to determine the volume of distribution (Vz) or clearance (CL).

6.9 Absolute bioavailability (F)

The absolute bioavailability refers to the proportion of a medicine that enters the systemic circulation following given by a route other than intravenous. In order for medications to be deemed appropriate for controlled-release drug delivery systems (CRDDS), it is desirable for the F value to exhibit a proximity to 100% [32].

6.10 Intrinsic absorption rate constant (Ka)

In order to ensure that the method of release is the rate-regulating step, it is normally necessary for the intrinsic absorption rate constant of the drug, when supplied orally in the form of a solution, to be significantly higher, typically by an order of magnitude, than the desired release rate constant of the drug from the dosage form [33].

6.11 Therapeutic concentration (Css)

The therapeutic concentrations encompass the desired or target steady-state peak concentrations (Css max), the desired or target steady-state minimum concentrations (Css min), and the mean steady-state concentration (Css avg). The distinction between CSS max and CSS min lies in the variability. The precision of the dosage form performance must be increased in order to achieve fewer desirable fluctuations. As the value of Css decreases, the magnitude of Vz decreases, resulting in an increase in the duration of t ½. Additionally, there is a corresponding increase in the magnitude of F. A smaller quantity of medication is necessary for integration into a controlled-release drug delivery system (CRDDS) [34].

7. Methods for creating controlled-release formulations

1. Controlled-release dissolution
    - Encapsulation dissolution control
    - Seed or granule coated
    - Micro-encapsulation
    - Matrix dissolution control
2. Diffusion controlled release
    - Reservoir-type devices
    - Matrix-type devices
3. Diffusion and dissolution controlled systems
4. Ion exchange resins
5. Osmotically controlled release

8. Factors affecting the design and implementation of controlled-release systems

8.1 Physiological properties

8.1.1 Aqueous solubility's

The majority of active pharmaceutical moieties (APIs) exhibit weak acidic or basic properties, which can impact the solubility of these APIs in water. Designing controlled-release formulations for weak water-soluble medicines might be challenging. Drugs with high solubility in aqueous solutions exhibit an initial burst release, which is thereafter followed by a rapid increase in the concentration of the drug in the plasma. These particular pharmaceutical compounds exhibit favorable characteristics that make them suitable candidates for controlled-release drug delivery systems (CRDDS). The solubility of CRDDS is problematic due to its dependence on pH. BCS class-III and class-IV medicines are deemed unsuitable candidates for this particular sort of formulations [35].

8.1.2 Partition coefficient (P-value)

The p-value represents the proportion of the drug that partitions into the oil and aqueous phases, which is a statistically significant factor influencing the passive diffusion of the medication across the biological membrane. The medications exhibit varying P values, which may not be conducive for controlled release (CR). Therefore, it is imperative that the drugs possess the ability to dissolve effectively in both aqueous and lipid phases [36].

8.1.3 Drug pKa

The pKa value is a critical determinant of the drug's ionization throughout the gastrointestinal tract at physiological pH. In general, medicines with high ionization are not considered suitable candidates for controlled-release drug delivery systems (CRDDS). The rate of absorption of unionized pharmaceuticals is significantly faster in comparison with ionized drugs while crossing biological membranes. The pKa range for an acidic medicine, whose ionization is pH-dependent, spans from 3.0 to 7.5. Conversely, the pKa range for a basic drug falls within the range of 7 to 11 [37].

8.1.4 Drug stability

Pharmaceutical substances that exhibit stability in acidic or basic environments, as well as resistance to enzymatic degradation and other gastric fluids, are considered favorable candidates for controlled-release drug delivery systems (CRDDS). If a medicine undergoes degradation in the stomach and small intestine, it is not considered ideal for controlled-release formulations due to the potential loss in bioavailability of the drug in question [38].

8.1.5 Molecular size and molecular weight

The molecular size and molecular weight are two critical variables that influence the diffusibility of molecules through a biological membrane. Molecules of a size below 400D exhibit a high degree of diffusibility, but those beyond 400D provide challenges in terms of drug diffusion [39].

8.1.6 Protein binding

The drug-protein combination functions as a reservoir inside the plasma, effectively retaining the drug. Pharmaceutical compounds exhibiting elevated levels of plasma protein binding are deemed unsuitable candidates for controlled-release drug delivery systems (CRDDS) due to the fact that protein binding serves to prolong the biological half-life. Therefore, there is no requirement to maintain the sustained release of the medicine.

8.2 Biological factors

8.2.1 Absorption

The consistency of both the rate and amount of absorption plays a crucial role in the formulation of controlled-release drug delivery systems (CRDDS). Nevertheless, the step that significantly restricts the rate of drug release is the liberation of the drug from the dosage form. In order to prevent dose dumping, it is recommended that the absorption rate be quick while the release rate should be controlled. There are several factors that influence the absorption of medicines, including water solubility, log P, and acid hydrolysis [40].

8.2.2 Biological half-life ($t_{1/2}$)

Typically, the drug exhibits a brief half-life, necessitating frequent administration, making it a viable choice for a controlled-release system. A pharmaceutical compound characterized by a prolonged half-life necessitates administration at extended intervals. Ideally, medicines with a half-life of 2–3 h are considered suitable candidates for controlled-release drug delivery systems (CRDDS). Pharmaceutical substances exhibit a half-life (t1/2) exceeding a duration of 7–8 h when not employed under a regulated release mechanism [41].

8.2.3 Dose size

The CRDDS was developed with the intention of reducing the need for repetitive dosing, necessitating the inclusion of a larger amount compared to standard dosage forms. However, the dosage employed in traditional dosage forms provides a reference for determining the appropriate dosage in controlled-release drug delivery systems (CRDDS). The magnitude of the sustained dose volume should be maximized to ensure compliance with the established acceptance criteria [42].

8.2.4 Therapeutic window

Drugs possessing a limited therapeutic index are deemed unsuitable for controlled-release drug delivery systems (CRDDS). In the event of a failure to regulate the release mechanism, it would result in dose dumping and subsequent toxicity as shown in **Figure 3.**

8.2.5 Absorption window

Pharmaceutical compounds that exhibit absorption from a particular segment in the gastrointestinal tract (GIT) are not considered optimal candidates for

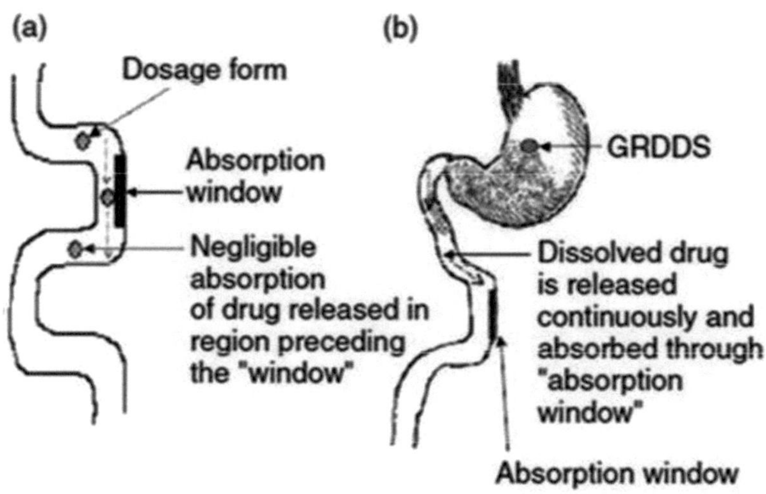

Figure 3.
Absorption pathway of drug delivery system.

Parameter	Comment
Elimination half-life	The recommended duration falls within the range of 2–6 h.
Elimination rate constant(KE)	Design is a fundamental requirement.
Total clearance (CLT)	Dose independent
Intrinsic absorption rate	It ought to be higher than the release pace
Apparent volume of distribution (Vd)	Vd affect the necessary dosage of the drug
Absolute bioavailability	75% or more
Steady state concentration (Css)	Less Css and lesser Vd
Toxic concentration	Therapeutic window must be widened

Table 1.
Pharmacokinetic parameters for drug selection.

controlled-release drug delivery systems (CRDDS). Pharmaceutical substances that undergo absorption within the gastrointestinal tract (GIT) exhibit favorable characteristics for controlled-release applications.

8.2.6 Patient physiology

The release of a drug from its dosage form is directly or indirectly influenced by the physiological condition of the patient, including factors such as gastric emptying rate, residence time, and gastrointestinal illnesses. The pharmacokinetic factors that are considered throughout the drug selection process are shown in **Table 1**.

9. Polymer used in controlled drug delivery system

The significance of polymers in medication delivery is progressively growing. Polymers find diverse applications in the field of pharmaceuticals, encompassing their utilization as binders in tablet formulations, as well as agents for controlling viscosity and flow in liquids, suspensions, and emulsions [43]. Polymers have the potential to serve as film coatings in order to mask the unpalatable flavour of pharmaceuticals, improve their stability, and alter their release properties. This review centers on the importance of pharmaceutical polymers in the context of controlled drug delivery applications. Currently, a significant number of individuals, estimated at sixty million, experience positive outcomes as a result of utilizing sophisticated drug delivery systems. These systems offer enhanced safety and efficacy in administering appropriate dosages of medications, hence aiding in the treatment of many human afflictions, such as cancer [44]. Controlled drug delivery (CDD) refers to the deliberate combination of a polymer, whether it is of natural or synthetic origin, with a drug or any other active agent. This combination is carefully planned to enable the release of the active ingredient from the material in a predetermined manner. The active agent's release can exhibit constancy, cyclic patterns, or be contingent upon environmental factors or external stimuli over an extended duration. The underlying objective of drug delivery regulation is to enhance the efficacy of medicines while mitigating the risks associated with both suboptimal and excessive doses [45].

10. Polymers as biomaterials for delivery systems

Various materials have been utilized for the purpose of regulating the release of pharmaceutical medicines and other bioactive substances. The initial development of these polymers mostly focused on nonbiological applications, driven by their advantageous physical characteristics.

- Poly(urethanes) were chosen for their flexibility,
- While poly(siloxanes) or silicones were selected for their insulating capabilities.
- Poly(methyl methacrylate) (PMMA) is a polymer that is widely recognized for its exceptional physical strength and transparency.
- Poly(vinyl alcohol) (PVA) is commonly utilized in various applications due to its desirable properties of hydrophilicity and strength.
- Poly(ethylene) is commonly used in various applications due to its desirable properties, such as toughness and resistance to swelling.
- On the other hand, poly(vinyl pyrrolidone) is often chosen for its ability to suspend particles effectively.

In order for a material to be effectively employed in formulations for controlled drug administration, it is imperative that the material possesses chemical inertness and is devoid of any leachable contaminants [46]. In addition, it is imperative for the entity to possess a suitable physical composition, characterized by little undesirable deterioration, and be easily amenable to processing. Several polymers are now employed for regulated drug delivery, including poly(2-hydroxy ethyl methacrylate), poly(N-vinyl pyrrolidone), and poly(methyl methacrylate). Poly(vinyl alcohol) is a polymer that is commonly used in various applications due to its unique properties. Poly(acrylic acid) is a polymer that is commonly used in various applications [47].

The following polymers will be discussed: polyacrylamide, poly(ethylene-co-vinyl acetate), poly(ethylene glycol), and poly(methacrylic acid).

Polymers, such as polyethylene, polyvinyl chloride, methyl acrylate, and ethylcellulose, are characterised by their insolubility and inertness [48].

The substances carnauba wax, stearyl alcohol, and castor wax are characterized by their insolubility and erodibility. The hydrophilic substances mentioned include methyl cellulose, hydroxyethyl cellulose, sodium carboxymethyl cellulose, and sodium alginate.

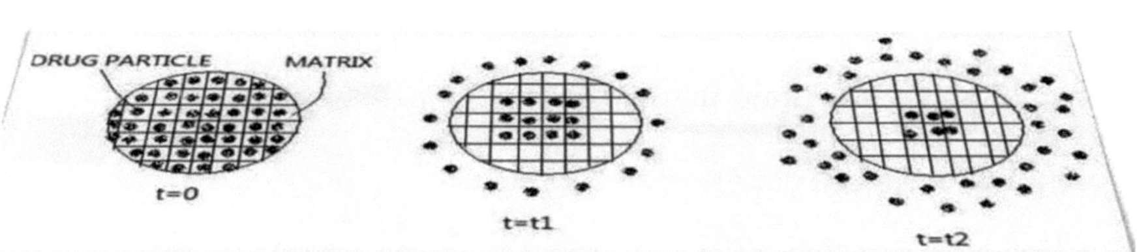

Figure 4.
Porous matrix composed of a water-insoluble polymer.

The medicine is distributed as solid particles within a porous matrix composed of a water-insoluble polymer, such as polyvinyl chloride, in a matrix system as shown in **Figure 4**.

At the onset, the drug particle situated on the surface of the release unit will undergo dissolution, leading to a fast release of the drug. Subsequently, drug particles located at progressively greater distances from the surface of the release unit will undergo dissolution and subsequently be released through diffusion through the pores, ultimately reaching the external environment surrounding the release unit [49]. The primary determinants influencing the release rate from a matrix system include the quantity of drug present inside the matrix, the porosity of the release unit, and the drug's solubility. In recent years, there has been an emergence of additional polymers specifically engineered for medicinal purposes, which have been relevant in the field of controlled release. A few of these materials have been specifically engineered to undergo degradation within the human body. A limited subset of these materials falls within this category [50].

- Polylactides (PLA).
- Polyglycolides (PGA).
- Poly(lactide-co-glycolides) (PLGA).
- Polyanhydrides.
- Polyorthoesters.

Initially, absorbable sutures were fabricated using polylactides and polyglycolides. Consequently, researchers naturally progressed to exploring the application of these polymers in the development of controlled drug delivery systems. One notable benefit of these degradable polymers is in their ability to undergo degradation into biologically acceptable compounds, which can subsequently be metabolized and eliminated from the body by regular metabolic processes. Nevertheless, it is important to acknowledge that biodegradable materials do generate breakdown by-products, which must be accepted within the biological environment without causing significant negative reactions [51].

Thorough testing of both desirable and potentially nondesirable degradation products is necessary, as several factors might influence the biodegradation of the initial materials. The below enumeration presents a comprehensive overview of the significant aspects that contribute to the extensive range of structural, chemical, and processing features that have the potential to influence biodegradable drug delivery systems [52].

- Chemical structure
- Distribution of repeat units in multimers
- Presence of unexpected units or chain defects.
- Molecular weight.
- Morphology (amorphous/semi-crystalline, microstructures, residual stresses).

- Presence of low-molecular-weight compounds.
- Sterilization process.
- Site of implantation.
- Adsorbed and absorbed compounds (water, lipids, ions, etc.)
- Physicochemical factors (ion exchange, ionic strength, pH).

11. Applications of controlled drug delivery system

Controlled drug delivery systems in the pharmaceutical industry refer to technologies that allow for precise control over the rate, time, and place of drug release within the body. These systems have various applications, offering benefits such as improved efficacy, reduced side effects, and increased patient compliance. Here are some pharmaceutical applications along with examples [53–55]:

Oral Drug Delivery:

Extended-Release Tablets: These release the drug over an extended period, maintaining therapeutic levels and reducing dosing frequency. Example: OxyContin (oxycodone).

Gastric Retentive Systems: These systems ensure prolonged drug presence in the stomach, which can enhance absorption or provide a local effect. Example: Proton pump inhibitors like Dexilant (dexlansoprazole).

Colon-Specific Delivery: Utilized for drugs that need to reach the colon for local or systemic effects. Example: Asacol (mesalamine) for treatment of ulcerative colitis.

Transdermal Drug Delivery:

Patches: These deliver drugs through the skin at a controlled rate, offering prolonged systemic effects. Example: Nicotine patches for smoking cessation.

Topical Gels/Creams: Control the release of drugs for localized effects on the skin or underlying tissues. Example: Voltaren Gel (diclofenac) for pain relief.

Intravenous Drug Delivery:

Infusion Pumps: These systems deliver a constant and controlled infusion of drugs directly into the bloodstream. Example: Insulin pumps for diabetic patients.

Liposomes and Nanoparticles: These can encapsulate drugs, allowing for targeted delivery and controlled release. Example: Doxil (liposomal doxorubicin) for cancer treatment.

Intramuscular and Subcutaneous Injections:

Depot Injections: These release the drug slowly from an injected depot, providing sustained effects. Example: Risperdal Consta (risperidone) for schizophrenia.

Ocular Drug Delivery:

Sustained-Release Implants: These implants slowly release drugs into the eye for conditions like macular degeneration. Example: Ozurdex (dexamethasone implant).

Ophthalmic Inserts: These deliver drugs to the eye over an extended period. Example: Dextenza (dexamethasone insert) for postoperative pain and inflammation.

Pulmonary Drug Delivery:

Dry Powder Inhalers (DPIs): These deliver drugs to the lungs in a fine powder form for localized or systemic effects. Example: Advair Diskus (fluticasone/salmeterol) for asthma.

Nebulizers: These convert liquid medication into a mist that can be inhaled for respiratory conditions. Example: Pulmicort Respules (budesonide) for asthma.

Nasal Drug Delivery:

Nasal Sprays: These can provide controlled delivery of drugs for local or systemic effects. Example: Flonase (fluticasone propionate) for allergic rhinitis.

Intrauterine Devices (IUDs):

Hormonal IUDs: These release hormones for contraception over an extended period. Example: Mirena (levonorgestrel-releasing IUD).

Intraperitoneal Drug Delivery:

Chemotherapy: Intraperitoneal delivery can provide controlled release of chemotherapy drugs directly into the abdominal cavity for treating ovarian cancer.

Implantable Devices:

Drug-Eluting Stents: These are used to prevent restenosis (re-narrowing) of arteries after angioplasty. Example: Cypher Stent (sirolimus-eluting stent).

These examples demonstrate the diverse range of controlled drug delivery systems and their applications in the pharmaceutical industry, allowing for more precise and effective treatment options for various medical conditions [56, 57].

12. Discussion

Drugs and excipients are combined in the dose form. Excipients are used to give products structure, improve stability, and cover up their flavors. Conventional dosage forms like solid, semisolid, and liquid require high doses and frequent administration while having poor patient compliance due to variations in plasma drug levels. Any dose form must include a medicine that is bioavailable in order to have the desired effect. Controlled drug delivery systems have become a viable alternative to traditional methods for maintaining drug plasma levels within the therapeutic range while increasing bioavailability, extending drug release, and minimizing negative effects. Controlled drug delivery allows the selective release of medications with a predictable pace and mechanism, as well as increased drug solubility and stability [11].

The several kinds of controlled drug delivery systems include diffusion, water penetration, dissolution, and chemically controlled drug delivery systems. Delivery methods that respond to stimuli can be used to target and regulate the release of substances in a variety of illness situations, including cancer and infections. To further accomplish controlled targeted delivery, nanocarriers with intelligent biomaterials and additive manufacturing processes can be developed. Patient-specific therapy using microfluidic-based, 3D-printed devices, and CRISPR cas9-based delivery systems linked with quantum sensing are the main goals of drug delivery in the future [58].

13. Future prospects

The field of controlled-release technology is still being developed despite the numerous controlled-release appliances that have been studied and/or used recently. Significant improvements in medication research, together with improved and earlier preventive medicine diagnostics, have contributed to an increase in human life expectancy. As a result, more medications are needed to treat a variety of illnesses, including coronary artery disease, diabetes mellitus, chronic pain, chronic lower respiratory disease, Alzheimer's disease, and Parkinson's disease. The first and most crucial step is to find medications for these illnesses. Drug candidates with poor water solubility can be transformed into therapeutically useful drug formulations, while those with short half-lives can be transformed into formulations for sustained release. The advancement of novel medications will greatly benefit from the drug delivery technology.

To deliver medications with various distinct qualities, a variety of drug delivery methods must be devised. The evolution of medication delivery systems has resulted from many iterations and failures, or trials and errors. It is necessary to test a wide range of medication delivery methods and to iterate on the most promising ones. Until a suitable treatment for a condition is discovered, this procedure must continue. Instead of using the same strategy that others have been doing for a decade or more, it is necessary to try numerous other techniques. For instance, numerous nanoparticle-based medication delivery systems have been created, yet they all use essentially the same methodology and only have minor variations.

It should be emphasized once more that the aim of research into medication delivery systems is to create patient-friendly formulations. Clear objectives are necessary for the development of efficient drug delivery systems. A new delivery method alone is insufficient. It must be safe and effective when used inside the human body. Clinical applications have some limitations, and it is important to get those out of the way early on in the development process. Understanding the characteristics of the drug delivery systems as well as biological barriers is the foundation for developing therapeutically viable drug delivery systems, which many mistakenly refer to as solving practical difficulties. In terms of drug distribution, there is no such thing as a "basic study" and a "practical study." Only the study of creating clinical formulations to treat different ailments exists.

Consent for publication

Not Applicable.

Conflict of interest

The author confirms that this chapter contents have no conflict of interest.

Author details

Muhammad Saeed Jan[1*], Waqas Alam[2] and Madeeha Shabnam[3]

1 Department of Pharmacy, Bacha Khan University, Charsadda, KP, Pakistan

2 Department of Pharmacy, Abdul Wali Khan University, Mardan, KP, Pakistan

3 Department of Chemistry, Women University, Mardan, KP, Pakistan

*Address all correspondence to: saeedjan@bkuc.edu.pk

References

[1] Maiti S, Sen KK. Introductory chapter: Drug delivery concepts. Advanced Technology Delivered Therapy. 2017;**26**:1-12

[2] Mostafavi E, Medina-Cruz D, Vernet-Crua A, Chen J, Cholula-Diaz JL, Guisbiers G, et al. Green nanomedicine: The path to the next generation of nanomaterials for diagnosing brain tumors and therapeutics? Expert Opinion on Drug Delivery. 2021;**18**(6):715-736

[3] Li N, Sun C, Jiang J, Wang A, Wang C, Shen Y, et al. Advances in controlled-release pesticide formulations with improved efficacy and targetability. Journal of Agricultural and Food Chemistry. 2021;**69**(43):12579-12597

[4] Dave PN, Macwan PM. Advanced fiber materials in drug delivery. In: Fiber Materials: Design, Fabrication and Applications. New York: Wiley; 2023. p. 273

[5] Hwang D, Ramsey JD, Kabanov AV. Polymeric micelles for the delivery of poorly soluble drugs: From nanoformulation to clinical approval. Advanced Drug Delivery Reviews. 2020;**156**:80-118

[6] Qiu Y, Lee P. Rational design of oral modified-release drug delivery systems. In: Developing Solid Oral Dosage Forms. Netherlands: Elsevier Inc; 2017. pp. 519-554

[7] Zhou QT, Leung SSY, Tang P, Parumasivam T, Loh ZH, Chan H-K. Inhaled formulations and pulmonary drug delivery systems for respiratory infections. Advanced Drug Delivery Reviews. 2015;**85**:83-99

[8] Bermejo M, Sanchez-Dengra B, Gonzalez-Alvarez M, Gonzalez- Alvarez I. Oral controlled release dosage forms: Dissolution versus diffusion. Expert Opinion on Drug Delivery. 2020;**17**(6):791-803

[9] Gajdošová M, Vetchý D, Muselík J, Gajdziok J, Juřica J, Vetchá M, et al. Bilayer mucoadhesive buccal films with prolonged release of ciclopirox olamine for the treatment of oral candidiasis: In vitro development, ex vivo permeation testing, pharmacokinetic and efficacy study in rabbits. International Journal of Pharmaceutics. 2021;**592**:120086

[10] Hoque J, Bhattacharjee B, Prakash RG, Paramanandham K, Haldar J. Dual function injectable hydrogel for controlled release of antibiotic and local antibacterial therapy. Biomacromolecules. 2018;**19**(2):267-278

[11] Adepu S, Ramakrishna S. Controlled drug delivery systems: Current status and future directions. Molecules. 2021;**26**(19):5905

[12] Shirin VA, Sankar R, Johnson AP, Gangadharappa H, Pramod K. Advanced drug delivery applications of layered double hydroxide. Journal of Controlled Release. 2021;**330**:398-426

[13] Kamaly N, Yameen B, Wu J, Farokhzad OC. Degradable controlled-release polymers and polymeric nanoparticles: Mechanisms of controlling drug release. Chemical Reviews. 2016;**116**(4):2602-2663

[14] Gardenhire DS, Burnett D, Strickland S, Myers T. Aerosol Delivery Devices for Respiratory Therapists. Irving, TX: American Association for Respiratory Care; 2017

[15] Tiwari R. Controlled release drug formulation in pharmaceuticals: A study on their application and properties. World Journal of Pharmaceutical Research. 2016;**5**:1740-1720

[16] Anand O, Pepin XJ, Kolhatkar V, Seo P. The use of physiologically based pharmacokinetic analyses—in biopharmaceutics applications-regulatory and industry perspectives. Pharmaceutical Research. 2022;**39**(8):1681-1700

[17] Deshpande A, Rhodes C, Shah N, Malick A. Controlled-release drug delivery systems for prolonged gastric residence: An overview. Drug Development and Industrial Pharmacy. 1996;**22**(6):531-539

[18] Madan J, Pandey RS, Jain V, Katare OP, Chandra R, Katyal A. Poly (ethylene)-glycol conjugated solid lipid nanoparticles of noscapine improve biological half-life, brain delivery and efficacy in glioblastoma cells. Nanomedicine: Nanotechnology, Biology and Medicine. 2013;**9**(4):492-503

[19] Borman AM, Fraser M, Palmer MD, Szekely A, Houldsworth M, Patterson Z, et al. MIC distributions and evaluation of fungicidal activity for amphotericin B, itraconazole, voriconazole, posaconazole and caspofungin and 20 species of pathogenic filamentous fungi determined using the CLSI broth microdilution method. Journal of Fungi. 2017;**3**(2):27

[20] Eschenauer G, DePestel DD, Carver PL. Comparison of echinocandin antifungals. Therapeutics and Clinical Risk Management. 2007;**3**(1):71-97

[21] Xia P, Verhey LJ. Multileaf collimator leaf sequencing algorithm for intensity modulated beams with multiple static segments. Medical Physics. 1998;**25**(8):1424-1434

[22] Senthilkumar S. Development of Polymer based Controlled Drug Delivery Systems of Selected Antibacterial Agents. Chennai: The Tamilnadu Dr. MGR Medical University; 2014

[23] Baggot JD. The Physiological Basis of Veterinary Clinical Pharmacology. New York: Wiley; 2001

[24] Kleinstreuer C. Biofluid Dynamics: Principles and Selected Applications. CRC Press; 2006

[25] Bandopadhyay S, Bandyopadhyay N, Deb PK, Singh C, Tekade RK. Preformulation studies of drug substances, protein, and peptides: Role in drug discovery and pharmaceutical product development. In: Dosage Form Design Considerations. Netherlands: Elsevier Inc; 2018. pp. 401-433

[26] Vree T, Muskens A, Van Rossum J. Some physico-chemical properties of amphetamine and related drugs. The Journal of Pharmacy and Pharmacology. 1969;**21**(11):774-775

[27] du Souich P. Absorption, distribution and mechanism of action of sysadoas. Pharmacology & Therapeutics. 2014;**142**(3):362-374

[28] Liebner R, Mathaes R, Meyer M, Hey T, Winter G, Besheer A. Protein HESylation for half-life extension: Synthesis, characterization and pharmacokinetics of HESylated anakinra. European Journal of Pharmaceutics and Biopharmaceutics. 2014;**87**(2):378-385

[29] Jødal L, Brøchner-Mortensen J. Reassessment of a classical single injection 51Cr-EDTA clearance method for determination of renal function in children and adults. Part I: Analytically correct relationship between total and one-pool clearance. Scandinavian Journal

of Clinical and Laboratory Investigation. 2009;**69**(3):305-313

[30] Mager DE, Jusko WJ. General pharmacokinetic model for drugs exhibiting target-mediated drug disposition. Journal of Pharmacokinetics and Pharmacodynamics. 2001;**28**:507-532

[31] Ghafourian T, Barzegar-Jalali M, Dastmalchi S, Khavari-Khorasani T, Hakimiha N, Nokhodchi A. QSPR models for the prediction of apparent volume of distribution. International Journal of Pharmaceutics. 2006;**319**(1-2):82-97

[32] Perucca E, Bialer M. Critical aspects affecting cannabidiol oral bioavailability and metabolic elimination, and related clinical implications. CNS Drugs. 2020;**34**:795-800

[33] Perez-Ruixo C, Rossenu S, Zannikos P, Nandy P, Singh J, Drevets WC, et al. Population pharmacokinetics of esketamine nasal spray and its metabolite noresketamine in healthy subjects and patients with treatment-resistant depression. Clinical Pharmacokinetics. 2021;**60**:501-516

[34] Gowda BJ, Ahmed MG, Alshehri SA, Wahab S, Vora LK, Thakur RRS, et al. The cubosome-based nanoplatforms in cancer therapy: Seeking new paradigms for cancer theranostics. Environmental Research. 2023;**237**:116894

[35] Anwar MKM, Sarode RS, Sonune AG, Sayyad ST, Kute MVG. A review on controlled release drug delivery system. 2023

[36] Debotton N, Garsiani S, Cohen Y, Dahan A. Enabling oral delivery of antiviral drugs: Double emulsion carriers to improve the intestinal absorption of zanamivir. International Journal of Pharmaceutics. 2022;**629**:122392

[37] Gaohua L, Miao X, Dou L. Crosstalk of physiological pH and chemical pKa under the umbrella of physiologically based pharmacokinetic modeling of drug absorption, distribution, metabolism, excretion, and toxicity. Expert Opinion on Drug Metabolism & Toxicology. 2021;**17**(9):1103-1124

[38] Zhou D, Porter WR, Zhang GG. Drug stability and degradation studies. In: Developing Solid Oral Dosage Forms. Netherlands: Elsevier Inc; 2017. pp. 113-149

[39] Chen S-S, Taylor JS, Mulford LA, Norris CD. Influences of molecular weight, molecular size, flux, and recovery for aromatic pesticide removal by nanofiltration membranes. Desalination. 2004;**160**(2):103-111

[40] Saha P, Das PS. Advances in controlled release technology in pharmaceuticals: A review. World Journal of Pharmaceutical Sciences. 2017;**6**(9):2070-2084

[41] Podust VN, Balan S, Sim B-C, Coyle MP, Ernst U, Peters RT, et al. Extension of in vivo half-life of biologically active molecules by XTEN protein polymers. Journal of Controlled Release. 2016;**240**:52-66

[42] Zadbuke N, Shahi S, Gulecha B, Padalkar A, Thube M. Recent trends and future of pharmaceutical packaging technology. Journal of Pharmacy & Bioallied Sciences. 2013;**5**(2):98

[43] Langer R. Polymer-controlled drug delivery systems. Accounts of Chemical Research. 1993;**26**(10):537-542

[44] Wu J, Zhang Z, Zhou W, Liang X, Zhou G, Han CC, et al. Mechanism of a long-term controlled drug release system based on simple blended electrospun fibers. Journal of Controlled Release. 2020;**320**:337-346

[45] Zhang A, Jung K, Li A, Liu J, Boyer C. Recent advances in stimuli-responsive polymer systems for remotely controlled drug release. Progress in Polymer Science. 2019;**99**:101164

[46] Idumah CI. Emerging advancements in xerogel polymeric bionanoarchitectures and applications. JCIS Open. 2022;**9**:100073

[47] Manzoor A, Dar AH, Pandey VK, Shams R, Khan S, Panesar PS, et al. Recent insights into polysaccharide-based hydrogels and their potential applications in food sector: A review. International Journal of Biological Macromolecules. 2022;**213**:987-1006

[48] Mansour D-EA, Abdel-Gawad NM, El Dein AZ, Ahmed HM, Darwish MM, Lehtonen M. Recent advances in polymer nanocomposites based on polyethylene and polyvinylchloride for power cables. Materials. 2020;**14**(1):66

[49] Tamani F, Bassand C, Hamoudi M, Danede F, Willart J-F, Siepmann F, et al. Mechanistic explanation of the (up to) 3 release phases of PLGA microparticles: Diprophylline dispersions. International Journal of Pharmaceutics. 2019;**572**:118819

[50] Sharma D, Dev D, Prasad D, Hans M. Sustained release drug delivery system with the role of natural polymers: A review. Journal of Drug Delivery and Therapeutics. 2019;**9**(3-s):913-923

[51] Graf TP, Qiu SY, Varshney D, Laracuente ML, Euliano EM, Munnangi P, et al. A scalable platform for fabricating biodegradable microparticles with pulsatile drug release. Advanced Materials. 2023;**35**:2300228

[52] Saboo S, Mugheirbi NA, Zemlyanov DY, Kestur US, Taylor LS. Congruent release of drug and polymer: A "sweet spot" in the dissolution of amorphous solid dispersions. Journal of Controlled Release. 2019;**298**:68-82

[53] Biondi M, Ungaro F, Quaglia F, Netti PA. Controlled drug delivery in tissue engineering. Advanced Drug Delivery Reviews. 2008;**60**(2):229-242

[54] Park W, Na K. Advances in the synthesis and application of nanoparticles for drug delivery. Wiley Interdisciplinary Reviews: Nanomedicine and Nanobiotechnology. 2015;**7**(4):494-508

[55] Scholz OA, Wolff A, Schumacher A, Giannola LI, Campisi G, Ciach T, et al. Drug delivery from the oral cavity: Focus on a novel mechatronic delivery device. Drug Discovery Today. 2008;**13**(5-6):247-253

[56] Ratnaparkhi MP, Gupta Jyoti P. Sustained release oral drug delivery system-an overview. Terminology. 2013;**3**(4):10-22270

[57] Smyth HD, Hickey AJ. Controlled Pulmonary Drug Delivery. Springer Science & Business Media; 2011

[58] Zhu Y, Bai Y, He J, Qiu X. Advances in the stimuli-responsive mesoporous silica nanoparticles as drug delivery system nanotechnology for controlled release and cancer therapy. 3 Biotech. 2023;**13**(8):274

Chapter 8

Importance of Nanoparticles in Cancer Therapy and Drug Delivery: A Detailed Theory and Gaps

Sagarkumar Patel and Rachna Patel

Abstract

Nanoparticles are a game-changing innovation in cancer therapy and drug delivery. Their ability to enhance drug targeting, overcome biological barriers, and minimize side effects makes them a cornerstone of modern oncology. The challenge lies in effectively distinguishing cancer cells from their regular counterparts in cancer therapy. Nanotechnology has emerged as a transformative solution, addressing this challenge through precise treatment modalities. This chapter delves into the pivotal role of Nanoparticles (NPs) in cancer therapy, primarily focusing on their significance in the drug delivery process. Overcoming the hurdles posed by conventional treatments, the genomic instability of tumors contributes to the variability among cancers, resulting in chemoresistance that challenges therapeutic success. A pioneering deep learning approach coupled with NPs has been proposed to tackle these issues, outshining previous methodologies by delivering drugs with accurate precision to target cancer cells and tissues. Through this innovative deep-learning technique, the proposed model achieves exceptional outcomes. With a remarkable accuracy of 97.591%, sensitivity of 96.644%, and specificity of 96.415%, the deep learning-enabled NPs demonstrate efficiency compared to the modern methods. This proposed model ushers in a new era of hope for patients and clinicians in the fight against cancer.

Keywords: deep learning, nanoparticles, drug resistance, cancer, nanotechnology, chemotherapy

1. Introduction

This section elaborates on the contemporary fusion of Nanotechnology and Artificial Intelligence in cancer therapy while elucidating the challenges inherent in diverse cancer treatments and the gamut of NPs employed in such therapeutic endeavors. The World Health Organization (WHO) estimates cancer's dire impact, ranking it the second dominant cause of global human mortality, accounting for approximately 10 million annual deaths [1]. This generic term encompasses a broad spectrum of diseases relentlessly afflicting the human body, often leading to fatal outcomes. In neoplasms, cancers manifest as uncontrolled proliferation of infected cells, potentially invading healthy neighboring cells, rendering the disease refractory

IntechOpen

to treatment. Accumulation beyond cell limits or avoidance of programmed cell death characterizes cancer, affecting various body parts. Cancers are broadly categorized as benign and malignant. Benign cancers grow slowly with distinct borders, while malignant cancers transgress boundaries, infiltrating adjacent cells. Carcinoma, sarcoma, leukemia, and lymphoma are prominent cancer types, further subcategorized based on origin. Early detection significantly improves prognosis, with indicative signs like fatigue, lumps, unexplained weight loss, skin changes, and persistent coughing. Breast cancers (BC) exemplify an aggressively metastatic variant, posing substantial therapeutic challenges [2]. Hormone therapy's ineffectiveness drives patients toward systemic chemotherapy, yet non-specific drug diffusion post-administration produces undesirable toxic effects. Multidrug resistance stemming from impaired drug intake and augmented drug efflux compounds these challenges, necessitating the development of effective BC treatments.

1.1 Nano technology

Nanotechnology presents an exact avenue for directing therapeutic agents to specific cancer cells and tissues, proficiently ferrying chemotherapy, radiotherapy, and immunotherapy drugs to their intended destinations. Extensive research has contributed to the creation of targeted nanocarriers aimed at controlling the release of antitumor drugs. Leveraging the enhanced permeation and retention (EPR) effect, investigators have formulated diverse NP platforms, including liposomes, polymer NPs, dendrimers, and so on, to transport anti-cancer agents into tumor tissues. Nonetheless, the effect of EPR alone does not suffice to eliminate cytotoxic drug side effects and ensure accurate anti-cancer drug delivery to cancer cells [3]. To augment targeting precision and uptake efficiency, NPs' external surfaces are often adorned with various ligands, significantly enhancing interactions between nanocarriers and cancer cells. These ligands encompass targeted agents such as antibodies, peptides, and small molecule compounds like folic acid. The recent past has witnessed extensive exploration of controlled drug delivery systems in the anti-cancer domain. An ideal drug delivery system must possess stability to retain loaded anti-cancer drugs during bloodstream circulation or in normal tissues. Both passive and active targeting mechanisms come into play for effective drug targeting and accumulation within tumor tissues. Once taken up by cancer cells, immediate drug release in response to the local environment is crucial [4]. The adaptability and responsiveness of stimulation-responsive polymer NPs have found widespread utility in tumor cell targeting, given their capacity to adjust to the tumor microenvironment.

1.2 Significance of therapy

Numerous cancer treatments have been developed, yet many have not realized their full potential in saving lives, underscoring the persistent global challenge of discovering innovative cancer therapies. Current cancer treatment modalities encompass a range of options involving surgery, chemotherapy, radiation therapy, immunotherapy, and so on. However, the lack of precise targeting of tumor cells undermines the efficacy of cancer treatments. Moreover, the necessity for higher drug doses to reach specific target cells often results in toxic effects within the human body. While chemotherapy is a widely employed cancer treatment method globally, it presents challenges. Its mechanisms for eliminating malignant cells also affect healthy cells, resulting in serious repercussions such as bone marrow suppression, hair loss, and gastrointestinal issues [2]. Thus, the central focus of numerous research endeavors in cancer treatment lies in developing therapies that target tumor cells without harming healthy cells, aiming to alleviate these treatment-associated concerns.

Chemotherapy treatment uses potent chemicals to halt the growth of tumors by delivering anti-cancer drugs directly to them [2]. It is effective against fast-growing cancer cells due to their quicker replication. Immunotherapy harnesses the body's natural defense system and enhances the immune response to identify and eliminate cancer cells. It can be used alone or combined with other treatments like chemotherapy. Biomarker testing involves analyzing genes, proteins, and other substances unique to an individual's cancer to tailor treatment approaches. Drugs are developed based on the specific biomarker pattern of the cancer. Biomarker testing involves analyzing genes, proteins, and other substances unique to an individual's cancer to tailor treatment approaches. Drugs are developed based on the specific biomarker pattern of the cancer. By manipulating hormones, this Hormone Therapy treatment restricts tumor growth. It can involve suppressing, blocking, or adding particular hormones to the body. Radiation therapy destroys cancer cells by using intense radiation beams, often X-rays and laser beams. Proton radiation is also employed to target cancer cells effectively. A cancer surgery involves removing tumors from the body, occasionally necessitating the removal of adjacent healthy tissue to control cancer spread [2].

1.3 Role of artificial intelligence in cancer therapy

Artificial Intelligence enabled by deep learning furnishes the vision-based technologies and prediction of patterns utilized in cancer therapy. In the particular area of bioinformatics, deep models can detect complex patterns in medical datasets to produce accurate insights and predictions. In biomedical imaging, deep learning is applied for several tasks, such as segmentation of tumor-affected tissue imaging [5]. For example, the tumor-affected blood cells can be predicted by employing a modified CNN architecture to target the cells to assist the NPs loaded with anti-cancer drugs to inhibit the cancer. Other models focus on easing data collection, and often, deep CNNs are trained for cell segmentation to formulate labeled datasets automatically utilizing fluorescently labeled cells. Hence, the most significant problem of deep learning models is the requirement for large annotated datasets to be collected by experts. To eliminate this problem, artificial NPs datasets are created, accelerating the data collection by forming annotated datasets without requiring expert manual annotations. Finally, in association with the object reconstruction, incorporating NPs for cancer targeting and deep models assisted the sophisticated systems that further classified the cancer and determined the complex disease patterns. Additionally, AI techniques help in biomarker detection, predicting interactions of NPs with the targeted drug, and evaluating drug efficacy.

1.4 Role of NPs in cancer therapy

Nanotechnology has emerged as the best solution for various medical applications due to its capability to deal with the dimensions and tolerances of less than 100 nanometers specifically for tackling individual molecular sizes [6]. Nanotechnology offers the exact approach to delivering the drugs into the target cells and tissues. With the assistance of these tools, medical experts can effectively transfer chemotherapy, radiotherapy, and immunotherapy drugs into the infected cells of the human body [7]. NPs are tiny elements that have size ranges from 1 to 100 nm. These NPs are categorized into multiple classes based on their shapes, sizes, and properties. The different types of NPs include metal NPs, ceramic NPs, and polymeric NPs. Additionally, the NPs possess specific properties because of high surface area and nano-scale size [8]. The physical properties relevant to the size and different colors are observed due to the absorption of NPs in the visible region [9]. Hence, the physiochemical properties enabled the NPs to be employed in medical applications like cancer treatment.

1.4.1 Types of NPs for cancer therapy

1.4.1.1 Organic NPs

Organic NPs are formed with the configuration of organic molecules that are virtually infinite numbers of unique structures or polymers. These organic materials are used in wide applications due to the ease of fabrication and the wide range of amassed structures that furnish better biocompatibility and biodegradation that make them suitable for drug delivery [10–12]. Additionally, the organic NPs provided antitumor efficacy and improved bioavailability compared to other NPs. Some organic NPS include dendrimers, polymeric NPS, liposomes, nanoemulsions, etc.

Polymeric NPs, structured through diverse monomers, range from 1 to 1000 nm [13]. They can encapsulate or adsorb active substances within their polymeric core for drug delivery. These hyperbranched NPs [14] have adjustable branches, aiding nucleic acid-targeting. Examples include polyamidation, with sizes ranging from 1 to 10 nm. Monoclonal antibody NPs, forming antibody-drug conjugates, precisely target cancer cells [15]. Paclitaxel core with a modified surface enhances efficiency and reduces toxicity. Extracellular Vesicles (EVs): From 50 to 1000 nm, EVs are lipid vesicles discharged by cells, like exosomes, macrovesicles, and apoptotic bodies. Exosomes penetrate cancer cells, delivering cytotoxic drugs. Spherical vesicles encapsulate drugs with a hydrophilic core and phospholipid bilayer. Low toxicity and inertness characterize liposomes. Cyclodextrin Nano sponges: These tiny NPs enhance drug loading, stabilizing and solubilizing agents like camptothecin drugs within cyclodextrin-based nanosponges.

1.4.1.2 Inorganic NPs

While compared with organic NPs, inorganic NPs possess the merits of maximum surface area to volume ratio and are safe as well as biocompatible and stable [6]. The most commonly used inorganic NPs involve gold NPs, carbon nanotubes, quantum dots, and magnetic NPs.

a. **Carbon NPs**: These are carbon-based NPs widely employed for their optical and electronic properties and biocompatibility. These NPs encapsulate the drugs through π-π stacking due to their hydrophobic nature. Carbon NPs include graphene, fullerenes, carbon nano horns, etc.

b. **Quantum Dots**: The quantum dots are semiconductors with a broad spectrum of absorption and narrow emission bands that make them applicable to biological imaging. The graphene quantum is utilized highly in drops because of their high intrinsic biocompatibility and discharge.

c. **Metallic NPs** are highly investigated in biological imaging and targeted in cancer cells because of their extraordinary optical, magnetic, and photothermal properties [13]. Generally utilized metallic NPs are silver NPs, iron-based NPs [16], gold NPs, and so on. Moreover, gold NPs are employed for intracellular targeting due to their tiny size and surface coating. The silver NPs (Ag NP) stimulated the ROS generation that inhibited the ATP synthesis and destroyed the cancer cells without damaging the healthy cells, as the normal cells are more resistant to cancer therapies.

d. **Magnetic NPs**: These are typically used in MRI imaging and as a carrier for drugs comprising metal and metal oxides and are enveloped with polymers and fatty acids to improve stability and compatibility. Magnetic NPs are also employed for targeted cancer therapy like magnetic hyperthermia, gene therapy, and controlled drug delivery [17–19].

e. **Calcium Phosphate NPs**: These are biologically compatible, biodegradable, and non-toxic, making them suitable for the delivery of antibiotics, growth factors, etc. Calcium phosphate can be combined with viral and non-viral vectors as carriers for gene transfer [20].

f. **Silica NPs**: Silica NPs are employed for delivering the genes by formulating the surface coating with amino-silicanes and are broadly used in immunotherapy due to minimal toxicity [21, 22].

1.4.1.3 Hybrid NPs

Hybrid NPs are high-potential heat transfer NPs acquired from suspending two or more dissimilar NPs in a regular heat transfer liquid [6]. Due to the high heat transfer properties of hybrid NPs, integrated different NPs advantages are widely used in industrial, manufacturing, and biomedical imaging processes [18].

a. **Lipid-polymer hybrid**: These are NPs comprising polymer cores and lipid/lipid-PEG shells that reveal the contrast characteristics of liposomes and polymeric NPs, uniquely in terms of their stability and biocompatibility [6, 15, 23].

b. **Organic-inorganic hybrid**: These hybrid NPs merge the variability of organic materials with the profiles often associated with inorganic materials. Hybrid NP comprises a silica core with an encapsulating lipid bilayer and is synthesized and validated in transferring the drugs to destroy the prostate and breast cancer cells [21, 24–26].

c. **Cell membrane coating hybrid**: These hybrid NPs are synthesized to rectify cancer. Cell membranes are derived from multiple natural cells and forced to encapsulate around different NPs to activate the immune response and targeting mechanism [27].

1.4.2 Synthesis of NPs

Multiple synthesis methods are adopted according to the different shapes, sizes and properties of the NPs [28–31]. The forms are categorized into two groups that include the approaches as follows.

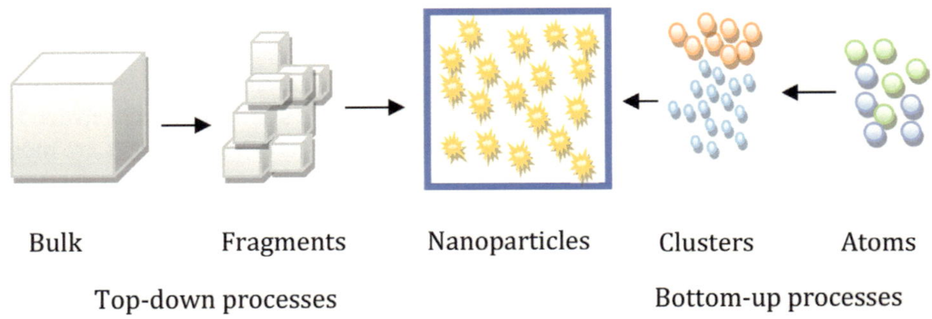

Figure 1.
Synthesis of NPs with top-down and bottom-up techniques.

1.4.2.1 Bottom-up approach

The method concerns building materials from atoms to clusters and further to NPs, which is the process of building the NPs from simpler particles, otherwise known as the constructive approach [13]. The generally employed techniques include spinning, sol–gel synthesis, vapor deposition, flame spraying, etc. (**Figure 1**).

1.4.2.2 Top-down approach

This method is also known as a destructive approach that depletes the heavy materials to synthesize the NPs. The more giant molecules are reduced into small blocks and converted into NPs [13]. The methods involve milling, nanolithography, laser ablation, and so on. Additionally, the characteristics related to the structure can be altered by changing the condition and other synthesized parameters. An in-depth knowledge of growth mechanisms is required for synthesizing the NPs.

1.4.3 Drug resistance operation

The drug resistance exhibited by tumor cells is a significant drawback of conventional therapies in cancer treatment, where the genomic instability aids the tumor to identify the heterogeneity between the cancers that progress the drug resistance of cancer cells [32]. The cancer cells acquire resistance to the drugs as the genes encoding the sequence of amino acids of proteins develop the mutation that can tolerate the changes according to the drugs injected in the tumor cells. The drug resistance mechanism includes the factors responsible for the drug resistance, such as efflux transporters, apoptosis process, and hypoxia response [33–36].

1.4.3.1 Focused approach to P-gp efflux transporter targeting

The efflux transporters reduce the drug accumulation by forcing the drugs out of the tumor cell, causing therapy failure. Glycoprotein is the most observed efflux transporter [23]. The high level of P-gp efflux transporters results in the inefficient treatment of the cancer [32]. The lipid phase of the plasma membrane plays a significant role in drug resistance as lipids can influence the proteins inside the plasma membrane by the membrane thickness. The membrane thickness affects the drug delivery, which can be reduced by combination therapy where the drugs are assembled within a single NP for drug delivery [37–39].

1.4.3.2 Targeting the process of apoptosis

The reactive oxygen species (ROS) formation in the mitochondria destroys the proteins, cell membranes, and DNA through the process of apoptosis, and the defective apoptosis process causes drug resistance in tumor cells [32]—the apoptosis process influenced by the lipids involved in the process. The drug-resistance cells preserve intracellular ceramide levels by enhancing the sphingomyelinase synthesis or reducing SM breakdown. Additionally, Adriamycin-resistant maintained ceramide level by multiplying the copies of an enzyme that converts ceramide to anti-apoptotic. Hence, combined therapies can be adopted to eliminate drug resistance in such conditions [40].

1.4.3.3 Targeting hypoxia response

Hypoxia is the situation determined at which the tumor cells are found with deprived oxygen levels. As a tumor grows, it requires a high blood supply, leaving portions where the oxygen concentration is reduced with the healthy cells. Hence, the enhanced interaction between the ceramide molecules forms the phase separation. The cells slowly multiplied in the hypoxic areas and avoided with cytotoxic drugs like alkylation agents and antibiotics [32]. The combined chemo-immunotherapy drugs delivery into perforated silicon NPs effectively stimulate the activation, cytotoxicity, and immune response against cancer cells.

2. Literature review

This section reviews recent methods, motivating the researchers to form the remarkable contributions of cancer therapy enabled by the deep learning model.

Anton Cid-Mejias et al. [5] developed a deep learning approach for segmenting the NPs in cancer therapy where the annotated datasets are created, followed by two CNNs for detecting and segmenting the NPs with their orientation. Finally, the reconstruction detected the shape of the nanoparticles utilized in the therapy. The approach does not require the annotated database and is adaptable but focused on the generated data validation.

Lei Liu et al. [14] developed a deep learning technique for analyzing the cytotoxicity of the Ag NPs where the decision tree is utilized in the model to facilitate the binary classification of the data and different combinations of features were extracted that provided the details involving the size, extraction solvent, exposure dose, and exposure time of NPs in cancer therapy were evaluated. The ensemble methods involving the random forest and the decision tree were utilized for the multi-classification of the NPs. However, these attributes do not accurately classify cytotoxicity, as the characteristics of silver NPs are complex to compute.

Yang Shen et al. [41] suggested an SVM classification for cancer therapy in which the gene expression data is utilized for the diagnosis. The method where the elastic net and fused lasso provided the smoothness and oriented features were selected automatically, reducing the time consumption. However, the technique has low reliability, and the complexity of the model should be minimized.

Alexandros Laios et al. [42] developed the k-NN classifier for cytotoxic prediction in cancer therapy, where the nearest neighbors are determined by the intake variables, and the average growth is predicted. The optimum neighbors were evaluated based on error calculation. The method provided the feasibility using the k-NN approach and outperformed the logistic regression while the value of k increased, causing the overfitting problems.

Aman Chandra Kaushik et al. [43] developed an optimized deep neural network for evaluating the growth receptor bound with gold NPs for cancer therapy. The approach where the mutational details of the receptor units utilized in the method were retrieved furnished insights for the cancer cell targeting and proved the efficiency of the gold NPs in inhibiting the growth factor receptor by the synergistic effect against the growth factor. Finally, the drug delivery efficiency of the gold NPs for smooth targeting of the cancer cells was determined.

Yousef Nademi et al. [44] suggested a deep learning method for non-viral vector anti-cancer drug delivery. The approach where the Polyethyleneimine NPs with anticancer drug siRNA are transferred to the cancer cells by utilizing the deep classifiers including the random forest, perceptron, and regression network. The approach in which the average prediction value is computed from the decision tree. Then, the perceptron and random forest better predicted the target cells due to the non-linearity that stated that the chemical descriptors would further facilitate better drug delivery into the cancer cells.

Huimin Zhu et al. [45] developed the simulation of anti-cancer drugs utilizing the machine learning model where the Fuzzy inference system employed in the approach that split the evaluated data for training and testing that further analyzed the solubility of the busulfan in the supercritical carbon dioxide. The fuzzy inference integrated the grid partitioning technique for providing the accurate processing parameters that drive the solvent solubility in the medium. However, the model's reliability should be further improved in the method.

Min Li et al. [46] developed the deep model approach for drug sensitivity detection in cancer therapy. The method where the genomic features and information related to the chemicals in drug constituency was integrated and analyzed using the modified deep model known as Deep DSC that predicted the sensitivity of the cancer lines. The Deep DSC method provided the advantages of interpolating the unknown drug sensitivity values and fewer extrapolating errors. However, the model's root mean square values of leave one tissue out and compound out values are less.

Challenges:

- Most cancer therapies observe the challenges in drug resistance exhibited by the tumor cells, where the genomic instability of the tumor provides the heterogeneity between the cancers that progress the chemoresistance of cancer cells [14].

- However, the attributes, including the size, extraction solvent, exposure dose, and exposure time, do not accurately classify Ag NPs cytotoxicity as the characteristics of silver NPs are complex to compute and should be improved [14, 32].

- The deep learning method utilizing the k-NN classifier for cancer diagnosis performed the logistic regression. At the same time, the value of k increased, which caused the overfitting problems that caused the error in the accurate prediction of cancer cells [42].

- The major drawback of the complexity associated with cancer treatment is cancer's metastatic nature, which causes errors in the prediction models enabled with the deep learning methods [44].

The cancer therapies in the former methods with their merits and demerits are elaborated in Section 2, and the deep learning enabled NPs for cancer therapy are enumerated in Section 3. The performance and analysis of proposed deep learning-enabled NPs for cancer therapy are elaborated in Section 4, and the conclusion is depicted in Section 5.

3. Proposed deep learning enabled NPs for cancer therapy

3.1 Deep convolutional neural network (DCNN)

DCNN is a sub-type of neural network that takes the merits of the spatial structure of the inputs for predicting the cancer cells by segmenting the cancer cells from the healthy cells. CNN models comprise the stacked convolutional layers and pooling layers, where each pooling layer is located after a convolutional layer. When applied to cancer prediction, CNNs can automatically acquire prominent features from the input data comprising the cancer and healthy cells and detect the patterns associated with the cancer cells that assists the NPs in accurately targeting the cancer cells for delivering the drugs in the targeted cells. CNN provided the segmentation of tumor cells by creating ground truth labeled datasets, thereby reducing the annotation requirement. The convolution layers learn the features of the cancer cells from the trained instances. They are utilized for predicting the cancer cells from the normal cells that are further processed, enabling the deep learning allowed NPs to target the tumor cells for delivering the drugs. CNN was employed for segmentation of the cancer cells from the microscopic images where the white blood cells affected with cancer can be determined by the CNN model for prominent targeting by NPs.

3.2 Targeting mechanism of Nps enabled with deep learning in cancer therapy

Deep CNN can learn the hierarchical representation of the data that overcame the recent methods as they optimize the filters to acquire the characteristic features from images. Hence, the deep CNN used to predict cancer cells enables the NPs to target the cancer cells. NPs are a non-toxic and effective approach for cancer diagnosis, anti-cancer drug delivery, and treatment. The combined NPs with chemotherapy drugs are injected into the infected cells for cancer treatment. NPs can deliver the insoluble drugs into the confined and distant tumor sites while protecting the drugs from being released prematurely. Hence, the nanoparticles eliminate the side effects associated with conventional therapy techniques. NPs are selected based on their size, surface coating, and other chemical properties for effective drug delivery [32]. NPs target the mitochondria that synthesize adenosine triphosphoric acid (ATP) that is required to replicate the cancer cells. The NPs combination of anti-cancer drugs promotes ROS generation in the mitochondria, destroying the mitochondrial proteins, cell membranes, and DNA strands replication through apoptosis that inhibits the cancerous cell multiplication [15, 21, 40, 47].

Often, it is observed that the Ag NPs that stimulated the ROS generation inhibited the ATP synthesis and destroyed the cancer cells without any damage to the healthy cells, as the normal cells are more resistant to the cancer therapies.

3.3 Targeting through passive means

Passive targeting depends on the EPR effect, where the targeting is exhibited during the hypoxia condition or the inflammation as the endothelium layers become more permeable during the neovascularization period [13]. While the hypoxia condition exists, the growing tumor cells utilize more perforated blood vessels as they possess more holes, thereby causing the permeability of the blood vessels. Additionally, the blood vessels become less resistant to extravasations, allowing the NPs to get diffused within the blood vessels and accumulate within the tumor cells. The primary factor responsible for cell replication is the glycolysis process that causes the tumor environment to be acidic due to low pH, and this period can be utilized to release the anti-cancer drugs encapsulated with the pH-sensitive NPs targeting the tumor cells (**Figure 2**) [47].

3.4 Active targeting

Active targeted NPs deliver a certain quantity of drugs to targeted tumor cells within a particular organ in the body. Drug-loaded NPs, along with ligands, are utilized for identification by receptors on cancer cells to eliminate the non-specific distribution of drugs in the entire body cells and eliminate cytotoxicity and impacts of drugs on healthy cells and organs that it is impossible in traditional chemotherapy [32]. Active targeting highly relies on ligands like folate that bind to the receptors over the surface layers of tumor cells. NPs with ligands furnish the retention and accumulation of drugs in the target cells. The mechanism involves the identification of ligands by the target receptors on the tumor surface that differentiate

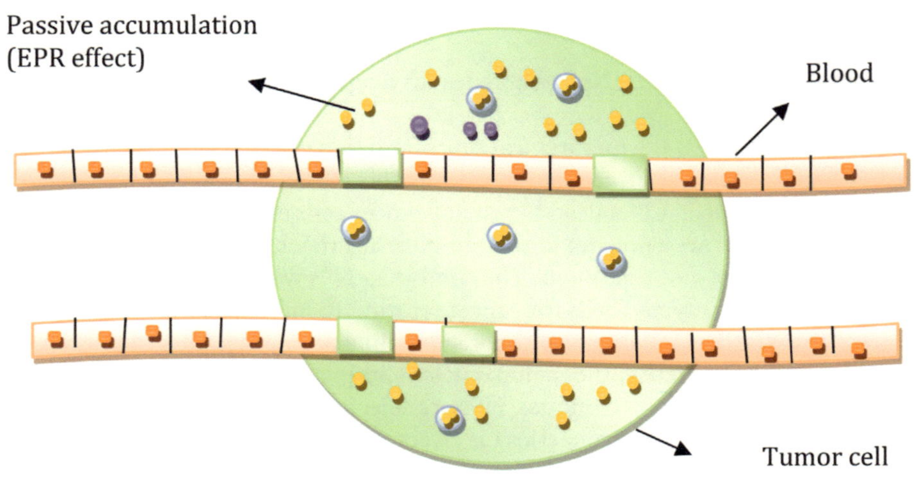

Figure 2.
Passive targeting.

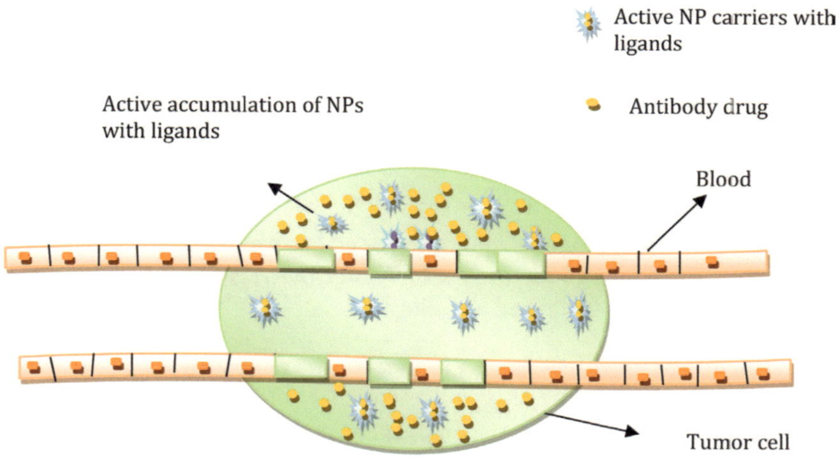

Figure 3.
Active targeting.

the tumor cells from the healthy cells. The ligands like peptides, antibodies, nucleic acids, vitamins, and so on can bind with the NPs and actively target the cancer cells (**Figure 3**).

4. Results and discussion

The proposed deep learning framework enabled with NPs for cancer therapy is executed, and the model outcomes are enumerated in the section to reveal the model's efficacy.

4.1 Experimental setup

The research is executed in Python, which comprises several programming methods; for instance, efficient programming and configuration of a system for the implementation involves PyCharm software running in the Windows 10 Operating System with 8GB internal RAM.

4.2 Dataset description

4.2.1 Breast cancer browse dataset

The datasets are collected from the breast cancer browse dataset in the UCI machine learning repository that contains multivariate images of about 286 instances with nine attributes for the validation testing and training of the deep models to provide efficient cancer diagnosis and cancer therapy utilizing the NPs [48].

4.2.2 SACT dataset

SACT datasets are collected from the SACT database organized by the Team of National Disease Registration Service (NDRS) at NHS England. It contains

44 data items that comprise the patient and tumor features, trust and consultant details, treatment characteristics, including drug specifications, and their combinations for training and testing of the datasets to provide efficient cancer therapy [49].

4.3 Performance analysis

The analysis of performance related to the deep learning-enabled NPs for cancer therapy is evaluated by employing the performance metrics, including the accuracy, sensitivity, and specificity described as follows.

4.3.1 Performance analysis for deep learning model enabled NPs for cancer therapy

The performance results of the deep learning helped NPs for cancer therapy, considering different epoch values, are depicted in **Figure 4**. In **Figure 4(a)**, the accuracy outcomes for TP 90, using the deep learning model, are as follows: 94.56%, 95.07%, 96.14%, 96.14, and 97.21% for epoch values of 100, 200, 300, 400, and 500, respectively. Correspondingly, **Figure 5(b)** displays the sensitivity values for TP 90, where the deep learning model achieves 94.77%, 95.12%, 95.85%, 95.85%, and 96.58% for epoch values of 100, 200, 300, 400, and 500, respectively. Likewise, **Figure 5(c)** shows cases of specificity over TP 90. The deep learning model demonstrates specificity values of 91.21%, 92.13%, 94.07%, 94.07%, and 96.01% for epoch values of 100, 200, 300, 400, and 500, respectively.

4.4 Comparative analysis

The comparative analysis of the deep learning enabled by NPs and different competent methods for cancer therapy is evaluated by employing the performance metrics described as follows.

4.4.1 Comparative analysis for deep learning model enabled NPs for cancer therapy

The comparative evaluation is estimated, and the result is acquired in terms of metrics depicted in **Figure 5**, in which the accuracy of the proposed method at TP 90 is 97.59%, which is enhanced by 8.5% to the former method D_1, 2.77% to D_2, 5.54% to D_3, 6.104% to D_4, 7.88% to D_5, and 8.55% to D_6. Moreover, the sensitivity at TP 90 is valued as 96.64%, which is progressed by 5.85% from the former method D_1, 5.39% from D_2, 11.25% from D_3, 4.17% from D_4, 3.79% from D_5 and 1.901% from D_6 as well as the specificity rate is 96.41% at TP 90 which is further progressed by 15.88% than D_1, 14.64% than D_2, 11.32% than D_3, 10.29% than D_4, 5.15% than D_5 and 3.09% than D_6 correspondingly. The analysis validated that the performance of the deep learning model is superior to the former methods. The systematic depiction of the comparative evaluation is demonstrated in **Figure 5**.

4.5 Comparative discussion

The evaluation of the deep learning-enabled NPs technique is enclosed in detail. Random Forest, KNN classifier, CATboost classifier, BiLSTM classifier, and deep CNN classifier are the former techniques employed for comparative evaluation. The

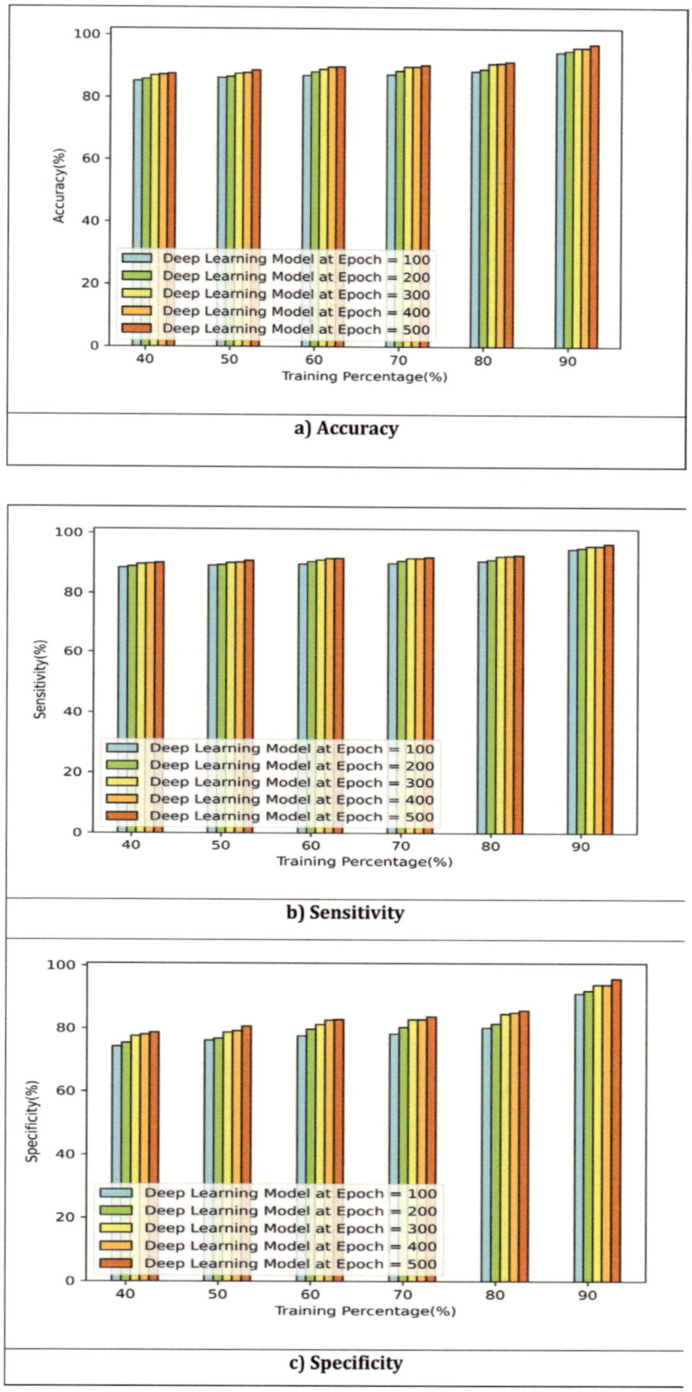

Figure 4.
Performance analysis for the proposed deep learning enabled NPs for cancer therapy.

performance of the enhanced classifiers at the early estimation of cancer is depicted here. **Table 1** represents the relative discussions of the deep learning-enabled NPs model with several existing systems.

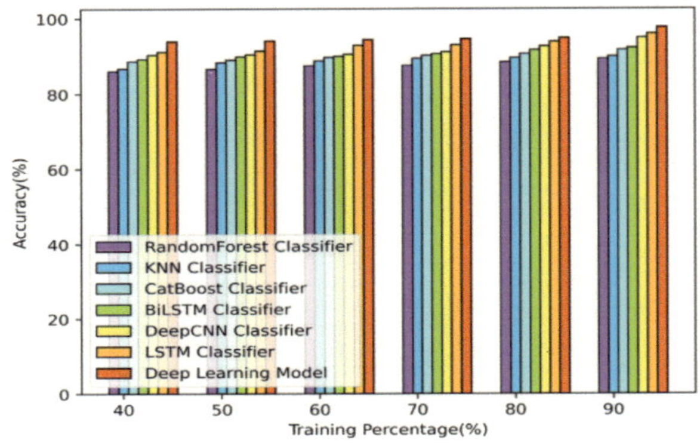

a) Accuracy

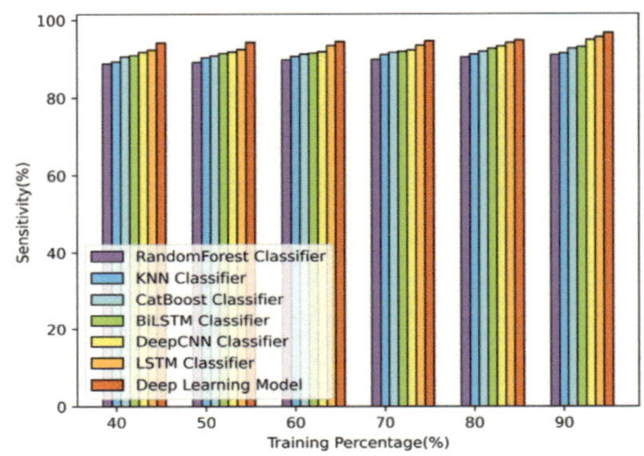

b) Sensitivity

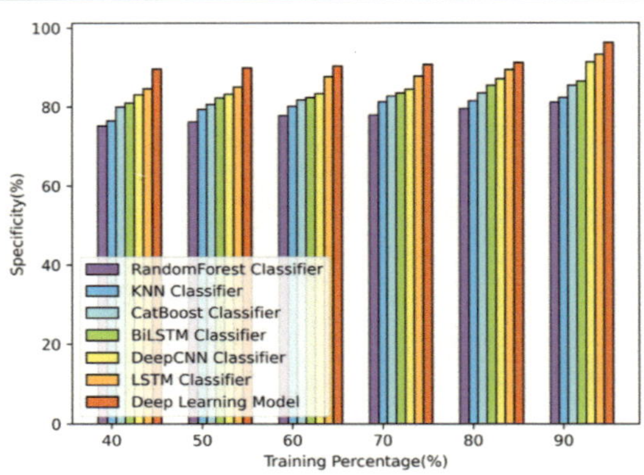

c)Specificity

Figure 5.
Comparative analysis of the proposed method: a) accuracy, b) sensitivity, c) specificity.

Methods	Training Percentage (%)		
	Accuracy	Sensitivity	Specificity
Random Forest D_1	89.273	90.983	81.101
KNN classifier D_2	89.891	91.426	82.302
Catboost classifier D_3	91.633	92.606	85.493
BiLSTM Classifier D_4	92.177	92.975	86.491
Deep CNN classifier D_5	94.879	94.807	91.445
LSTM Classifier D_6	95.963	95.542	93.433
Proposed Deep learning enabled NP model	97.591	96.644	96.415

Table 1.
Comparative discussion.

4.6 Applications

Deep learning algorithms integrate diverse data sources such as gene expression data (X), patient clinical data (C), and molecular characteristics (M). These inputs are analyzed to create a comprehensive patient profile (P), which captures crucial information about the patient's condition. Using the patient profile (P), a deep learning model predicts the optimal therapeutic strategy (T). This strategy involves selecting suitable therapeutic agents, dosages, and administration schedules tailored to the patient's specific characteristics. Deep learning generates nanoparticle design parameters (N) based on the therapeutic strategy (T). Parameters include attributes like the type of drug, optimal dosage, and selection of targeting ligands that enhance nanoparticle specificity to cancer cells. A deep learning model determines the efficiency of nanoparticles' targeting (TE). This model considers the expression of specific biomarkers (B) on cancer cells to calculate targeting efficiency. The eq. $TE = f(B)$ captures this relationship. The release profile of therapeutic agents from nanoparticles (R) is modeled through deep learning algorithms. PH (pH) and temperature (T) influence the release kinetics. The eq. $R = g\ (pH, T)$ characterizes the payload release process. Imaging data (I) obtained from techniques like MRI provides real-time feedback on the distribution of nanoparticles within the tumor.

Deep learning models analyze this data to assess and visualize the spatial distribution and effectiveness of treatment. Deep learning models utilize patient-specific data (P) to predict the likely treatment response (TR). Factors such as patient history, molecular characteristics, and treatment specifics contribute to predicting how the patient will respond to therapy. The eq. $TR = h(P)$ captures this prediction. As the patient progresses through treatment, new patient data (P_new) is continuously fed into the deep learning model. This adaptive approach ensures that the therapeutic strategy (T) is dynamically adjusted based on evolving patient characteristics, maximizing treatment efficacy. Deep learning models provide clinicians with valuable insights (I), aiding them in making informed decisions about treatment adjustments and patient management. These insights contribute to an ongoing and collaborative treatment approach.

5. Conclusion

The proposed deep learning method enabled by NPs overcame the challenges of the former methods in precisely delivering drugs to the affected cancer cells. Further, the deep learning methods support the discrimination between the cancer cells and normal cells and address the problems associated with the conventional chemotherapy of NPs. The deep CNN is employed for predicting the cancer cells by detecting the cancer cell patterns that enabled the NPs to target the cancer cells prominently. This research specifically focuses on the significance of NPs in cancer therapy, particularly in the drug discovery process. The proposed deep learning method enabled by NPs overcame the challenges of drug resistance and provided an exact approach for drug delivery to the target cancer cells and tissues. The proposed deep learning method enabled with NPs delivered the performance of 97.591% accuracy, 96.644% sensitivity, and 96.415% specificity, which is more efficient when compared to the recent methods. Further, the method can be enhanced by utilizing other classifiers and augmentation methods.

Author details

Sagarkumar Patel[1*] and Rachna Patel[2]

1 LabCorp Drug Development Inc, Somerset, NJ, USA

2 Catalyst Clinical Research LLC, NC, USA

*Address all correspondence to: sagarpatel5391@gmail.com

References

[1] Ferlay J, Colombet M, Soerjomataram I, Parkin DM, Piñeros M, Znaor A, et al. Cancer statistics for the year 2020: An overview. International Journal of Cancer. 2021;**149**(4):778-789. DOI: 10.1002/ijc.33588

[2] Pourmadadi M, Eshaghi MM, Ostovar S, Mohammadi Z, Sharma RK, Paiva-Santos AC, et al. Innovative nanomaterials for cancer diagnosis, imaging, and therapy: Drug delivery applications. Journal of Drug Delivery Science and Technology. 2023;**82**:104357

[3] Huang Y. Targeting glycolysis for cancer therapy using drug delivery systems. Journal of Controlled Release. 2023;**353**:650-662

[4] Das CA, Kumar VG, Dhas TS, Karthick V, Kumar CV. Nanomaterials in anti-cancer applications and their mechanism of action-a review. Nanomedicine: Nanotechnology, Biology and Medicine. 2023;**47**:102613

[5] Cid-Mejías A, Alonso-Calvo R, Gavilán H, Crespo J, Maojo V. A deep learning approach using synthetic images for segmenting and estimating 3D orientation of nanoparticles in EM images. Computer Methods and Programs in Biomedicine. 2021;**202**:105958

[6] Dang Y, Guan J. Nanoparticle-based drug delivery systems for cancer therapy. Smart Materials in Medicine. 2020;**1**:10-19

[7] Jafari S, Derakhshankhah H, Alaei L, Fattahi A, Varnamkhasti BS, Saboury AA. Mesoporous silica nanoparticles for therapeutic/diagnostic applications. Biomedicine & Pharmacotherapy. 2019;**109**:1100-1111

[8] Rane AV, Kanny K, Abitha VK, Thomas S. Methods for synthesis of nanoparticles and fabrication of nanocomposites. In: Synthesis of Inorganic Nanomaterials. Durban: Woodhead Publishing; 2018. pp. 121-139

[9] Ziental D, Czarczynska-Goslinska B, Mlynarczyk DT, Glowacka-Sobotta A, Stanisz B, Goslinski T, et al. Titanium dioxide nanoparticles: Prospects and applications in medicine. Nanomaterials. 2020;**10**(2):387

[10] Pandit C, Roy A, Ghotekar S, Khusro A, Islam MN, Emran TB, et al. Biological agents for the synthesis of nanoparticles and their applications. Journal of King Saud University - Science. 2022;**34**(3):101869. DOI: 10.1016/j.jksus.2022.101869

[11] Khurana A, Tekula S, Saifi MA, Venkatesh P, Godugu C. Therapeutic applications of selenium nanoparticles. Biomedicine & Pharmacotherapy. 2019;**111**:802-812

[12] Ottoni CA, Simões MF, Fernandes S, Dos Santos JG, Da Silva ES, de Souza RF, et al. Screening of filamentous fungi for antimicrobial silver nanoparticles synthesis. AMB Express. 2017;**7**(1):1-0

[13] Gavas S, Quazi S, Karpiński TM. Nanoparticles for cancer therapy: Current progress and challenges. Nanoscale research letters. 2021;**16**(1):173

[14] Liu L, Zhang Z, Cao L, Xiong Z, Tang Y, Pan Y. Cytotoxicity of photosynthesized silver nanoparticles: A meta-analysis by machine learning algorithms. Sustainable Chemistry and Pharmacy. 2021;**21**:100425

[15] Mu J, Zhong H, Zou H, Liu T, Yu N, Zhang X, et al. Acid-sensitive PEGylated

paclitaxel prodrug nanoparticles for cancer therapy: Effect of PEG length on antitumor efficacy. Journal of Controlled Release. 2020;**326**:265-275

[16] Soetaert F, Korangath P, Serantes D, Fiering S, Ivkov R. Cancer therapy with iron oxide nanoparticles: Agents of thermal and immune therapies. Advanced Drug Delivery Reviews. 2020;**163**:65-83

[17] Fariq A, Khan T, Yasmin A. Microbial synthesis of nanoparticles and their potential applications in biomedicine. Journal of Applied Biomedicine. 2017;**15**(4):241-248

[18] Khan T, Ullah N, Khan MA, Nadhman A. Plant-based gold nanoparticles; a comprehensive review of the decade-long research on synthesis, mechanistic aspects, and diverse applications. Advances in Colloid and Interface Science. 2019;**272**:102017

[19] Hasan A, Morshed M, Memic A, Hassan S, Webster TJ, Marei HE. Nanoparticles in tissue engineering: Applications, challenges, and prospects. International Journal of Nanomedicine. 2018:5637-5655

[20] Khalifehzadeh R, Arami H. Biodegradable calcium phosphate nanoparticles for cancer therapy. Advances in Colloid and Interface Science. 2020;**279**:102157

[21] He H, Meng S, Li H, Yang Q, Xu Z, Chen X, Sun Z, Jiang B, Li C. Nanoplatforms based on GSH-responsive mesoporous silica nanoparticles for cancer therapy and mitochondrial-targeted imaging. Microchimica Acta 2021; 188:1-0

[22] Chen S, Greasley SL, Ong ZY, Naruphontjirakul P, Page SJ, Hanna JV, et al. Biodegradable zinc-containing mesoporous silica nanoparticles for cancer therapy. Materials Today Advances. 2020;**6**:100066

[23] Khan H, Mirzaei HR, Amiri A, Akkol EK, Halimi SM, Mirzaei H. Glyco-nanoparticles: New drug delivery systems in cancer therapy. In: Seminars in Cancer Biology. Vol. 69. Pakistan: Academic Press; 2021. pp. 24-42

[24] She S, Chen H, Ji W, Sun M, Cheng J, Rui M, et al. Deep learning-based multi-drug synergy prediction model for individually tailored anti-cancer therapies. Frontiers in Pharmacology. 2022;**13**:1032875

[25] Avanzo M, Stancanello J, Pirrone G, Sartor G. Radiomics and deep learning in lung cancer. Strahlentherapie und Onkologie. 2020;**196**:879-887

[26] Snow O, Lallous N, Ester M, Cherkasov A. Deep learning modeling of androgen receptor responses to prostate cancer therapies. International Journal of Molecular Sciences. 2020;**21**(16):5847

[27] Raj S, Khurana S, Choudhari R, Kesari KK, Kamal MA, Garg N, et al. Specific targeting cancer cells with nanoparticles and drug delivery in cancer therapy. In: Seminars in Cancer Biology. Vol. 69. India: Academic Press; 2021. pp. 166-177

[28] Eaton P, Quaresma P, Soares C, Neves C, De Almeida MP, Pereira E, et al. A direct comparison of experimental methods to measure dimensions of synthetic nanoparticles. Ultramicroscopy. 2017;**182**:179-190

[29] Priyadarsini S, Mukherjee S, Mishra M. Nanoparticles used in dentistry: A review. Journal of Oral Biology and Craniofacial Research. 2018;**8**(1):58-67

[30] Zhao D, Yu S, Sun B, Gao S, Guo S, Zhao K. Biomedical applications

of chitosan and its derivative nanoparticles. Polymers. 2018;**10**(4):462

[31] Sun T, Zhang YS, Pang B, Hyun DC, Yang M, Xia Y. Engineered nanoparticles for drug delivery in cancer therapy. Nanomaterials and Neoplasms. 2021:12320-12364

[32] Miranda RR, Sampaio I, Zucolotto V. Exploring silver nanoparticles for cancer therapy and diagnosis. Colloids and Surfaces B: Biointerfaces. 2022;**210**:112254

[33] Partin A, Brettin TS, Zhu Y, Narykov O, Clyde A, Overbeek J, et al. Deep learning methods for drug response prediction in cancer: Predominant and emerging trends. Frontiers in Medicine. 2023;**10**:1086097

[34] Chang JW, Ding Y, Tahir ul Qamar M, Shen Y, Gao J, Chen LL. A deep learning model based on sparse auto-encoder for prioritizing cancer-related genes and drug target combinations. Carcinogenesis. 2019;**40**(5):624-632

[35] Bychkov D, Linder N, Tiulpin A, Kücükel H, Lundin M, Nordling S, et al. Deep learning identifies morphological features in breast cancer predictive of cancer ERBB2 status and trastuzumab treatment efficacy. Scientific Reports. 2021;**11**(1):4037

[36] Wang S, Zhang H, Liu Z, Liu Y. A novel deep learning method to predict lung cancer long-term survival with biological knowledge incorporated gene expression images and clinical data. Frontiers in Genetics. 2022;**13**:800853

[37] Paskeh MD, Entezari M, Clark C, Zabolian A, Ranjbar E, Farahani MV, et al. Targeted regulation of autophagy using nanoparticles: New insight into cancer therapy. Biochemicals et Biophysica Acta (BBA)-Molecular Basis of Disease. 2022;**1868**(3):166326

[38] Peetla C, Vijayaraghavalu S, Labhasetwar V. Biophysics of cell membrane lipids in cancer drug resistance: Implications for drug transport and drug delivery with nanoparticles. Advanced Drug Delivery Reviews. 2013;**65**(13-14):1686-1698

[39] Huda S, Alam MA, Sharma PK. Smart nanocarriers-based drug delivery for cancer therapy: An innovative and developing strategy. Journal of Drug Delivery Science and Technology. 2020;**60**:102018

[40] Känkänen V, Fernandes M, Liu Z, Seitsonen J, Hirvonen SP, Ruokolainen J, et al. Microfluidic preparation and optimization of sorafenib-loaded poly (ethylene glycol-block-caprolactone) nanoparticles for cancer therapy applications. Journal of Colloid and Interface Science. 2023;**633**:383-395

[41] Shen Y, Wu C, Liu C, Wu Y, Xiong N. Oriented feature selection SVM applied to cancer prediction in precision medicine. IEEE Access. 2018;**6**:48510-48521

[42] Laios A, Gryparis A, DeJong D, Hutson R, Theophilou G, Leach C. Predicting complete cytoreduction for advanced ovarian cancer patients using nearest-neighbor models. Journal of Ovarian Research. 2020;**13**:1-8

[43] Kaushik AC, Wang YJ, Wang X, Kumar A, Singh SP, Pan CT, et al. Evaluation of anti-EGFR-iRGD recombinant protein with GOLD nanoparticles: Synergistic effect on antitumor efficiency using optimized deep neural networks. RSC Advances. 2019;**9**(34):19261-19270

[44] Nademi Y, Tang T, Uludağ H. Modeling uptake of Polyethyleneimine/short interfering RNA nanoparticles in breast cancer cells using machine

learning. Advanced Nano Biomed Research. 2021;**1**(10):2000106

[45] Zhu H, Zhu L, Sun Z, Khan A. Machine learning based simulation of an anti-cancer drug (busulfan) solubility in supercritical carbon dioxide: ANFIS model and experimental validation. Journal of Molecular Liquids. 2021;**338**:116731

[46] Li M, Wang Y, Zheng R, Shi X, Li Y, Wu FX, et al. Deep DSC: A deep learning method to predict drug sensitivity of cancer cell lines. IEEE/ACM Transactions on Computational Biology and Bioinformatics. 2019;**18**(2):575-582

[47] Li Y, Wang S, Song FX, Zhang L, Yang W, Wang HX, et al. A pH-sensitive drug delivery system based on folic acid-targeted HBP-modified mesoporous silica nanoparticles for cancer therapy. Colloids and Surfaces A: Physicochemical and Engineering Aspects. 2020;**590**:124470

[48] UCI Machine Learning Repository [Internet]. archive.ics.uci.edu. [cited 2023 Sep 5]. Available from: https://archive.ics.uci.edu/datasets?search=cancer

[49] Systemic Anti-Cancer Therapy (SACT) data set [Internet]. NDRS. [cited 2023 Sep 5]. Available from: https://digital.nhs.uk/ndrs/data/data-sets/sact

Chapter 9

Prospective Bacterial Minicells for Drug Delivery Systems

Nguyen Hoang Khue Tu

Abstract

Drug delivery system (DDS) is an important challenge in medicine over the conventional drug delivery system in case of therapeutic efficacy. In recent years, due to the shortcomings of conventional chemotherapy such as poor bioavailability, low treatment index, and unclear side effects, the focus of drug development and research has shifted to new nanocarriers of chemotherapeutic drugs. By using biodegradable materials, nanocarriers generally have the advantages of good biocompatibility, low side effects, specific target, controlled release profile, and improved efficacy. There are many kinds of DDS such as lyposome, vesicle, peptide, gene, microchip, polysaccharide and so on being studied nowadays. Each DDS has the advantages and disadvantage. However, the materials made them are expensive and the preparation techniques sometimes are complicated. Moreover, those DDS are rarely shown the ability in drug delivery to target. In the study, nano sized bacterial minicells were showed to clarify the importance of this material in drug delivery and target therapy.

Keywords: bacteria, minicells, interaction of minicell components and drugs, molecular docking, drug delivery systems, nanoparticles

1. Introduction

The drug is delivered via entering the body, traveling through the bloodstream to go to the target and then eliminating out of the body [1, 2]. DDS is oriented to limit unwanted effects in human pharmacology. DDS must be biodegradable in the body, suggesting that DDS should be researched and exploited from various materials to obtain high bioavailability toward the target from which the possibility of drug resistance and side effects will be reduced, in addition to carrying drugs. Lyposomes, peptides, vesicles, polysaccharides, aptamers, viruses, and DNA are much being researched. However, each DDS can bring drugs and especially toward the target is valuable. Furthermore, targeted DDS is developed to achieve a higher level of treatment due to the disease target specificity but reduce side effects. Nanoparticles can also accumulate in the healthy organ where they can cause side effects [3, 4]. Nanoparticles must be potential to the target of the body, control drug release, and dramatically increase the bioavailability of active compounds. Various materials have been used to prepare nanoparticles for drug delivery systems. Liposome, polymer and minicell conjugated drugs were taken the preclinical trials. The first biodegradable nanoparticles are developed for drug delivery with the properties of lipid membranes such as Doxil [5]. According to the US National Cancer Institute, nanoparticles are currently authorized for use in the global market, while the cost of these products is ten times higher than conventional treatments [6]. At present, the use of nano-sized particles derived from bacteria which are called minicells to encapsulate a wide range of different chemotherapeutic drugs is a new technology that specifically targets to receptors on disease cell surface via dual-specific antibodies coated on the minicells. Minicell loaders have been shown the apoptosis effects on tumor cells both *in vitro* and *in vivo* with high specificity when delivering drug [7]. Although minicell is still a new concept in DDS, the term of minicell is appeared in a number of patents around the world as well as through clinical trials. Minicells are small cells produced by bacteria that could play many roles in the development of agents to treat cancer [7, 8]. With a bacterial structure with different functional groups and holes in the cell wall, minicells can bind with many drugs including chemicals and antibodies to reach the most favorable destination for developing a DDS. This study aims to point out the minicells derived nanoparticles for DDS to suggest a new opportunity for prospective nanoparticle development for pharmaceutical science.

2. Well-known drug delivery systems

2.1 Advantages of well-known DDSs

There are many drugs that are effective for treating diseases, but side-effects are still problematic when crossing the barriers in the body, for example eye barrier, colon, and brain membrane due to the complex structure of barriers of eye, colon, and brain. DDS can be microelectromechanical (MEM)-based device, polymer matrix or gene delivery system. DDS can be developed using pH, enzyme, time, pressure-controlled delivery method [9]. In some cases of colon treatment, a hole in the membrane is covered by an enteric-coated polymer to prevent drug release in the upper gastrointestinal tract. Brain-targeted drug delivery has received increasing attention over the past decade. Many strategies have been developed to improve brain-targeted drug delivery by fabricating particle-based drug delivery systems. Despite impressive progress, drug delivery efficiency remains unsatisfactory. Recent advances in the field of microfabrication have made possible the development of controlled release systems for drug delivery. Drug delivery has achieved tremendous development over the past two decades, but regulating drug delivery to the brain is going on a daunting task. By using such highly specialized transport mechanisms, it is possible to efficiently mediate the penetration of the nanodrug delivery system into the brain. Surface functionalization of DDS and selection of suitable materials for their membranes play an important role in drug release kinetics. The release of a particular drug from DDS can be regulated by external or internal stimuli. The pH-responsive DDS can only release the drug in the area it targets. Several pH-responsive DDSs have been successfully engineered to deliver drugs in tumor tissues because tumor tissues have a different pH than healthy tissues [10]. The reduced environment of the cytoplasmic fluid of the cell relative to the body fluid becomes a stimulus for redox-sensitive DDS to release active substances only in the cytosol but not in the body fluid [11]. Magnetic NPs loaded with therapeutic agents can be guided, using an externally applied magnetic field, to a specific organ and stimulated to release the drug only at that location [12]. Nanotechnology was first defined in 1974 by Norio Taniguchi of Tokyo University of

Science, as the technique and technology for understanding and controlling matter at the length scale of about 1 to 100 nanometers [1]. Many nanomaterial preparations have significant potential applications for therapeutic drug delivery systems. Several nano-sized preparations such as liposomes, polymeric micelles and polymer drug conjugates have been developed *in vitro*, and several preclinical studies are underway [13, 14]. Properties including the size, surface charge, shape and density of surface-related targeting ligands could allow nanoparticles to evade renal clearance to reach cellular targets. Indicated cells in sufficient quantities, undergo active cellular uptake, and induce biological responses with minimal non-specific interactions [15]. The raw materials of nanoparticles are not only of biological origin such as lactic acid, dextran, phospholipids, lipids, carbon and chitosan but also of chemical origin such as polymers, silica and metals [16–18]. The nanodrugs currently approved for the treatment of cancer are mainly liposomal nanoparticles. They have their structural, physicochemical properties giving hope to patients. Additionally, the gene therapy field approved viral vector-based drugs of various designs and purposes such as cancer therapies. Currently, the three main vector strategies are based on adenoviruses, adeno-associated viruses, and lentiviruses that occured in clinical and preclinical processes for the past decades. However, there are still many challenges for drug targeting in cancer therapy [19].

2.2 Challenges of well-known DDSs

Undoubtedly, the controlled DDS presents an important challenge in medicine when compared with the conventional DDS in the case of therapeutic efficacy. Accordingly, there has been a search for drug delivery systems that enhanced activity for more drugs with fewer complications. Until now, there are very few reports on the effects of nanoparticles on the body. The long-term effects on our health are difficult to predict and understand. Nanocarriers can increase the stability of many anticancer drugs by integrating them into their structures, for example, the stability of doxorubicin has also been increased through its incorporation into liposomes [20]. Previous reports showed a beneficial effect on the long-term stability of DNA when the molecule was complexed into polymeric micelles [21, 22]. Furthermore, the nanoparticles are antibacterial agents but can also kill the good bacteria in the gut. In addition, DDSs using nanoparticles are more expensive to manufacture than traditional materials because of the many complex steps [18]. Consequently, it is difficult to scale up the production of nanoparticles leading to the limited production in the market and also causing to many risks due to their unknown side effects. Drug delivery using nanoparticles is increasingly popular and faces many challenges in pharmaceutical engineering. There are many reports on nanotoxicology, the potential negative effects of interactions between nanomaterials and biological systems. For example, naked quantum dots exhibit cytotoxicity by generating reactive oxygen species, leading to nuclear, mitochondrial, and plasma membrane damage [17]. For silica nanoparticles, concentrations above 0.1 mg/ml were found to be toxic, as demonstrated by decreased cell proliferation and availability [17]. The production of carbon nanotubes also induced the formation of reactive oxygen species, mitochondria dysfunction, lipid peroxidation, and changes in cell morphology. In addition, it has been reported that most cationic NPs can induce hemolysis and coagulation, while neutral and anionic NPs did not show toxicity [23, 24]. For hydrophobic drugs, their main limitation is their low solubility at the absorption site and poor biodegradability. The case of many common hydrophobic drugs is well illustrated by paclitaxel that have low oral bioavailability in conventional formulations but the activity increase when formulated in DDS like liposome [25–27]. However, DDS which can carry different kinds of drugs to the disease target are challenged. Therefore, finding out the potential DDS is essential. In this chapter, bacterial minicells that have nano size are focused to show its ability in drug delivery.

3. Minicells in drug delivery

3.1 Minicells generated by microorganisms

Minicells are the small cells in nano size that can be call nanoparticles. They are made from the membranes of mutant bacteria during cell division cycle. The term "minicells" refers to cells that contain RNA and proteins but only small amounts of chromosomal DNA, if any at all. The genetic and biochemical characterization of the minicells of *Escherichia coli* revealed that most were defective in the multiprotein system known as the Min system, which mediates the alignment correct arrangement of the middle cells of the cell division septum [28, 29]. In *Escherichia coli*, the three proteins which are MinC, MinD, and MinE, synergistically mediate the niche of the cell division machinery by inhibiting its growth at sites location other than the middle cell [30]. In *Escherichia coli*, fts is temperature-sensitive filament involving mutants and partition (par) mutants [31]. There are FtsZ, FtsA, FtsK, FtsQ, FtsL, FtsB, FtsW, FtsI, and FtsZ. FtsZ, a tubulin homolog which are the essential components of septal ring, called a Z-ring at potential division positions, where more division proteins are recruited to form the complete division [31]. In *Escherichia coli*, Min proteins rapidly migrate from one pole of the cell to the opposite pole, forming a bipolar inhibitory gradient that prevents assembly of the Z ring near the poles but allows FtsZ to stay at the poles near the middle of the cell. Min system is not dependent on nucleoid occlusion and forms anucleate cells which are chromosome segregation mutants. Otherwise, when Min system lacks in cells, nucleoid occlusion is not enough to direct Z-ring assembly. Consequently, the division occurs at any one of three potential division site, a chromosome less-minicell and a multinucleate filament are produced [32]. The minicell mutants in *Escherichia coli* were mapped to the *min loc*us which encodes MinC, MinD, and MinE [31]. In *Bacillus subtilis*, the Min system includes MinC, MinD, DivIVA and DivIVB which are different from *Escherichia coli*. *Bacillus subtilis* does not have MinE. DivIVA localizes from poles to midcell of division sites. DivIVA has some functions beyond that of involving MinCD location. Together with DivIVA, DivIVB also participate in minicell formation [33]. Both Gram-positive and Gram-negative bacteria can produce minicells. Minicells were also produced in *Lactobacillus acidophilus* [34] or by gene expressing the cell division inhibitor [35]. Gram-negative cell wall consists of lipopolysaccharide, O-specific side chains, outer membrane, peptidoglycan, periplasmic space, and porins. Gram-positive cell wall is composed peptidoglycans, teichoic acid, and periplasmic space. A peptidoglycan network can cover with a variety of substances. Teichoic acid is a linear polymer of polyols in the form of glycerol or various monosaccharides linked by phosphodiester bridges [36]. The polysaccharides associated with different drugs, antibodies and so on. Minicells with a uniform diameter around 400 nm were produced from both Gram-positive and Gram-negative bacteria. Based on bacterial properties, minicells can play a potential role in drug delivery (**Figure 1**).

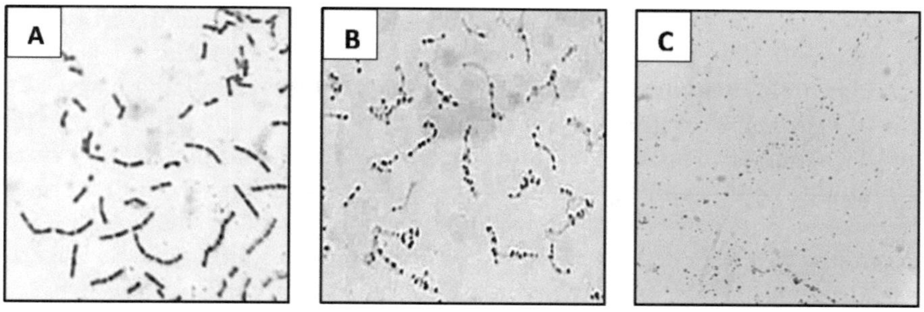

Figure 1.
Gram staining and observing Lactobacillus acidophilus. (A): Minicells started producing from rod cells in supplemented MRS medium in 36 hours. (B): Minicells produced from rod cells in supplemented MRS medium in 48 hours. (C): Purified Minicells.

3.2 Minicell loading with different drugs

Interestingly, minicells can be packed with 1–10 million drug molecules [17]. Minicells traverse tumor cells by receptor-mediated endocytosis. *In vivo* experiments, doxorubicin-loaded minicells inhibited tumor growth in mice such as breast, ovary, leukemia or lung [37]. Importantly, a relatively small amount of drug is needed to induce tumor regression, 100 times the higher dose required with liposome-encapsulated doxorubicin. The antitumor efficacy of minicells was further evaluated in dogs with end-stage T-cell non-Hodgkin lymphoma; treatment resulted in marked tumor regression and tumor lysis [38]. Importantly, multiple studies have shown that minicells have no adverse side effects despite repeated dosing and do not increase proinflammatory cytokines. Other animal experiments confirmed no adverse reactions [39]. Using microcells derived from bacteria for the first time used in humans with clear results is safe, well tolerated. Solomon reported that minicells encapsulated the chemotherapy drug paclitaxel and coated with antibodies targeting tumors that express an epidermal growth factor receptor (EGFR) protein found on the surface of many cancer cells. The study was then conducted in phase I for treating the small groups of patients. Phase II trials of minicells were continued in one group of patients with glioblastoma (a type of brain tumor) using doxorubicin-loaded minicells [39, 40]. *In vitro* studies, the small cells produced by *Lactobacillus* are nano-sized which are useful in drug delivery. *Lactobacillus* minicells can be loaded and reloaded with hydrophilic and hydrophobic drugs such as paclitaxel, cephalosporins without phagocytosis that suggested to one of valuable DDS [41]. There are many applications of minicells reported such as therapeutic research such as drug discovery, delivery of nucleic acids and other bioactive compounds to cells. MacDiarmid and colleagues described the use of chemotherapeutic-encapsulated bacterial small cells guided by antibodies to deliver their payloads to target cells by a recognized surface lipopolysaccharide dual-specific antibody (epidermal growth factor receptor (EGFR), HER2/neu (ERBB2), CD33 or CD3 [38].

By molecular docking application, different kinds of proteins of bacteria are expected to interact with a variety of ligands such as drugs. Molecular docking is a method to predict the drug molecule which can be bind to the proteins of the disease target based on a computation aid. In this study, protein-ligand concatenation was performed to see the ability of drugs in interacting with the target protein [42]. The 3D crystal structures of proteins from bacteria was obtained from the Protein Data Bank (PDB). Moreover, all the 3D structures of ligands like drugs were downloaded in Pubchem and ChemSpider [43]. Then, Autodock Vina were used to screen protein and ligand interaction, providing the binding affinity of each profile between the ligand and protein interactions. The Genetic Algorithm was calculated based on 10 runs for 10 different configurations of drugs to show the binding ability to the target protein [43]. Validation is based on Root Mean Standard Deviation (RMSD) value and the binding energy value (Kcal/mol) [44]. Interactions with amino acid residues in the receptor's active binding pocket were analyzed using BIOVIA Discovery Studio binding [45, 46]. The interactions between some proteins of *Escherichia coli*, *Salmonella enterica* subsp. enterica serovar Typhimurium, *Bacillus subtilis* with hydrophilic and hydrophobic drugs used as ligands were shown in **Table 1**. Maltose binding protein of *Escherichia coli* (ID: 3OSR), outer membrane protein A (OmpA) from *Salmonella enterica* subsp. enterica serovar Typhimurium (ID: 5VES), the outer membrane protein A and C (OmpA and C) of *Escherichia coli* (ID: 3NB3), *Escherichia coli* MinD (ID: 3Q9L), *Bacillus subtilis* N-terminal domain of MinC (ID 2M4I) could

Number	Proteins	Ligands	Binding energy (kcal/mol)
1	Maltose-bound maltose sensor engineered by insertion of circularly permuted green fluorescent protein into *Escherichia coli* O157:H7 maltose binding protein at position 311 (ID: 3OSR)	Vancomycin	−23.4
		Vincristine	−20.7
		Paclitaxel	−19.8
		Stigmasterol	−9.9
		Quercetin	−8.6
		Cephalexin	−7.7
		Ciprofloxacin	−7.7
		Erythromycin	−7.6
		Penicillin	−7.6
		Hydroxychloroquine	−7.4
2	The 2.4A crystal structure of OmpA domain of OmpA from *Salmonella enterica* subsp. enterica serovar Typhimurium str. 14028S (ID: 5VES)	Vancomycin	−19.1
		Vincristine	−17
		Vinblastine	−16.8
		Paclitaxel	−15.9
		Quercetin	−8
		Stigmasterol	−7.3
		Penicillin	−7
		Ciprofloxacin	−7
		Erythromycin	−6.9
		Cephalexin	−6.8
		Hydroxychloroquine	−5.9

Number	Proteins	Ligands	Binding energy (kcal/mol)
3	The host outer membrane proteins OmpA and OmpC are packed at specific sites in the *Shigella* phage Sf6 virion as structural components (ID: 3NB3)	Vancomycin	−21.6
		Vincristine	−17.3
		Vinblastine	−16.8
		Paclitaxel	−16.8
		Stigmasterol	−7.9
		Quercetin	−7.8
		Hydroxychloroquine	−5.7
		Erythromycin	−8.2
		Penicillin	−7
		Cephalexin	−7.3
		Ciprofloxacin	−7
4	The structure of the dimeric *Escherichia coli* MinD-ATP complex (ID: 3Q9L)	Paclitaxel	−19.7
		Vancomycin	−17.8
		Vinblastine	−14.7
		Vincristine	−14.6
		Erythromycin	−11.5
		Stigmasterol	−7.0
		Ciprofloxacin	−6.3
		Cephalexin	−6.2
		Quercetin	−6.1
		Penicillin	−5.7
		Hydroxychloroquine	−5.0
5	Solution structure of *Bacillus subtilis* MinC N-terminal domain (ID: 2M4I)	Vancomycin	−17.5
		Vincristine	−16.9
		Vinblastine	−15.9
		Paclitaxel	−13.1
		Erythromycin	−13.0
		Quercetin	−7.4
		Stigmasterol	−6.5
		Ciprofloxacin	−5.7
		Cephalexin	−5.3
		Penicillin	−5
		Hydroxychloroquine	−4.8

Table 1.
Interaction of some bacterial proteins with ligands using molecular docking.

bind to ligands with negative energy, showing the interaction. Depending on the protein and ligand, the binding ability was different.

As seeing in **Table 1**, beside outer membrane proteins could bind to drugs, cell division protein inhibitors such as MinC and MinD could interact to different drugs. **Figure 2** showed the representative studies of molecular docking for screening the interaction of MinD cell division inhibitor of *Escherichia coli* could bind to anticancer drug such as paclitaxel via hydrogen bond, Pi lone pair, Pi-sigma, Pi-anion, Pi-alkyl while vincrisrine interaction was by means of hydrogen bond, Pi-cation, Pi-alkyl, amide-Pi stacked (**Figure 2**). MinD protein could also bind to hydroxychloroquine, an antimalarial drug at the active sites which were Thr 17, Thr 18, Pro 212, Val 217, Glu213, and Arg 212 via the determined bonds (**Figure 2**). Besides, antibiotics such as erythromycin belonging to macrolide as well as cephalexin and penicillin belonging to beta-lactam group or alkaloids and steroids represented such as quercetin and stigmasterol could also bind to MinD that was illustrated in **Figure 2**. By these interactions, drugs/ligands can be released again from minicells when going to the target

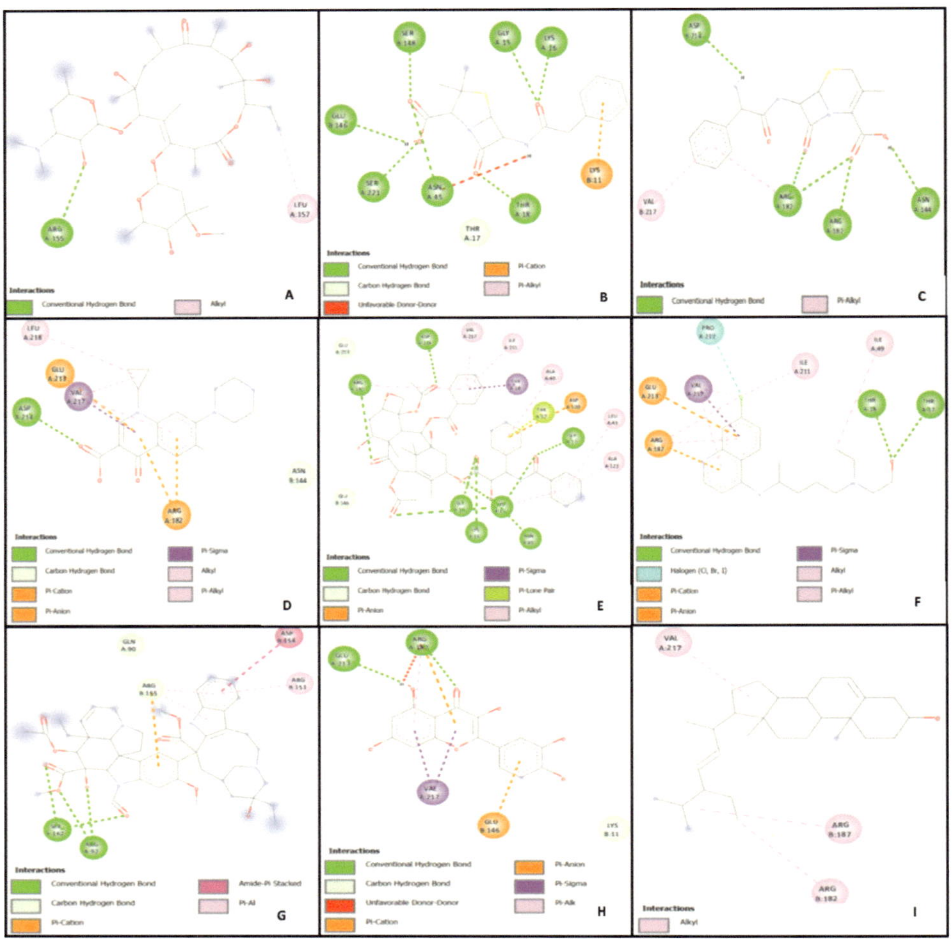

Figure 2.
Visualization of drugs with the highest binding energy interacts to MinD cell division inhibitor of Escherichia coli. (A): Erythromycin; (B): Penicillin; (C): Cephalexin; (D): CiproFloxacin; (E): Paclitaxel; F: Hydroxychloroquine; (G): Vincristine; (H): Quercetin; (I): Stigmasterol. (conventional hydrogen bond: Green color; pi-sigma bond: Purple color; pi-alkyl: Pink color; pi-cation: Orange colors).

sites. More studies will be developed for getting the ideal DDS. Therefore, with the structure of bacterial minicells, there are many kinds of drugs which can be bound to be delivered. As a result, bacterial minicells could be the potential drug delivery system for target treatment.

4. Conclusion

Nowadays, DDS is developed for targeting to therapy. With the small size like nanoparticle, the bioavailability of drugs increases. However, nanotechnology is still challenged. Some materials are not convenient for DDS development. Moreover, DDS which carries drug to the target to reduce side effect is very important for human health care. Bacterial minicells are cheap and can be produced in large scale. With the complexity of cell wall structure, minicells can bind with hydrophobic and hydrophilic drugs. Especially, minicells could bind to monoclonal antibodies which are specific to the target cells. Exploiting minicells give a good picture for cancer therapy, pathogen treatment and vaccine development.

Acknowledgements

The study was developed by private fund.

Conflict of interest

The authors declare no conflict of interest.

Author details

Nguyen Hoang Khue Tu[1,2]

1 School of Biotechnology, International University, Hochiminh City, Vietnam

2 Vietnam National University, Hochiminh City, Vietnam

*Address all correspondence to: nhktu@hcmiu.edu.vn

References

[1] Serda RE, Godin B, Blanco E, Chiappini C, Ferrari M. Multi-stage delivery nano-particle systems for therapeutic applications. Biochimica et Biophysica Acta. 2011;**1810**:317-329. DOI: 10.1016/j.bbagen.2010.05.004

[2] Wright J. Nanotechnology: Deliver on a promise. Nature. 2014;**509**:S58-S59. DOI: 10.1038/509S58a

[3] Davis ME, Chen Z, Shin DM. Nanoparticle therapeutics: An emerging treatment modality for cancer. Nature Reviews Drug Discovery. 2008;7:771-782. DOI: 10.1038/nrd2614

[4] Altammar KA. A review on nanoparticles: Characteristics, synthesis, applications, and challenges. Frontiers in Microbiology. 2023;**14**:1155622. DOI: 10.3389/fmicb.2023.1155622

[5] Barenholz Y. Doxil®–the first FDA-approved nano-drug: Lessons learned. Journal of Controlled Release. 2012;**160**(2):117-134. DOI: 10.1016/j.jconrel.2012.03.020

[6] Pillai G. Nanomedicines for cancer therapy: An update of FDA approved and those under various stages of development. SOJ Pharmacy & Pharmaceutical Sciences. 2014;**1**(2):13. DOI: 10.15226/2374-6866/1/1/00109

[7] MacDiarmid JA, Mugridge NB, Weiss JC, Phillips L, Burn AL, Paulin RP, et al. Bacterially derived 400 nm particles for encapsulation and cancer cell targeting of chemotherapeutics. Cancer Cell. 2007;**11**:431-445. DOI: 10.1016/j.ccr.2007.03.012

[8] MacDiarmid JA, Brahmbhatt H. Minicells: Versatile vectors for targeted drug or si/shRNA cancer therapy. Current Opinion in Biotechnology. 2011;**22**:909-916. DOI: 10.1016/j.copbio.2011.04.008

[9] Ramesh K, Sunit S, Pratibha S, Muralidharan J, Arun B, Anuj B. Randomized controlled trial comparing cerebral perfusion pressure–Targeted therapy versus intracranial pressure–Targeted therapy for raised intracranial pressure due to acute CNS infections in children. Critical Care Medicine. 2014;**42**(8):1775-1787. DOI: 10.1097/CCM.0000000000000298

[10] Ding H, Tan P, Fu S, Tian X, Zhang H, Ma X, et al. Preparation and application of pH-responsive drug delivery systems. Journal of Controlled Release. 2022;**348**:206-238. DOI: 10.1016/j.jconrel.2022.05.056

[11] Guo X, Cheng Y, Zhao X, Luo Y, Chen J, Yuan WE. Advances in redox-responsive drug delivery systems of tumor microenvironment. Journal of Nanobiotechnology. 2018;**16**(1):74. DOI: 10.1186/s12951-018-0398-2

[12] Schleich N, Po C, Jacobs D, Ucakar B, Gallez B, Danhier F, et al. Comparison of active, passive and magnetic targeting to tumors of multifunctional paclitaxel/SPIO-loaded nanoparticles for tumor imaging and therapy. Journal of Controlled Release. 2014;**194**:82-91. DOI: 10.1016/j.jconrel.2014.07.059

[13] Gaspar R, Duncan R. Polymeric carriers: Preclinical safety and the regulatory implications for design and development of polymer therapeutics. Advanced Drug Delivery Reviews. 2009;**61**:1220-1231. DOI: 10.1016/j.addr.2009.06.003

[14] Duncan R. Polymer therapeutics: Top 10 selling pharmaceuticals — What

next? Journal of Controlled Release. 2014;**190**:371-380. DOI: 10.1016/j.jconrel.2014.05.001

[15] Biswas S, Torchilin VP. Nanopreparations for organelle-specific delivery in cancer. Advanced Drug Delivery Reviews. 2014;**66**:26-41. DOI: 10.1016/j.addr.2013.11.004

[16] Dessale M, Mengistu G, Mengist HM. Nanotechnology: A promising approach for cancer diagnosis, therapeutics and theragnosis. International Journal of Nanomedicine. 2022;**17**:3735-3749. DOI: 10.2147/IJN.S378074

[17] De Jong WH, Borm PJA. Drug delivery and nanoparticles: Applications and hazards. International Journal of Nanomedicine. 2008;**3**:133-149. DOI: 10.2147/ijn.s596

[18] Singh R, Lillard JW. Nanoparticle-based targeted drug delivery. Experimental and Molecular Pathology. 2009;**86**:215-223. DOI: 10.1016/j.yexmp.2008.12.004

[19] Ghosh S, Brown AM, Jenkins C, Campbell K. Viral vector Systems for Gene Therapy: A comprehensive literature review of Progress and biosafety challenges. Applied Biosafety. 2020;**25**:7-18. DOI: 10.1177/1535676019899502

[20] Torchilin VP. Recent advances with liposomes as pharmaceutical carriers. Nature Reviews Drug Discovery. 2005;**4**:145-160. DOI: 10.1038/nrd1632

[21] Bashir SM, Ahmed Rather G, Patrício A, et al. Chitosan nanoparticles: A versatile platform for biomedical applications. Materials (Basel). 2022;**15**(19):6521. DOI: 10.3390/ma15196521

[22] Gary DJ, Puri N, Won Y-Y. Polymer-based siRNA delivery: Perspectives on the fundamental and phenomenological distinctions from polymer-based DNA delivery. Journal of Controlled Release. 2007;**121**:64-73. DOI: 10.1016/j.jconrel.2007.05.021

[23] Bamrungsap S, Zhao Z, Chen T, Wang L, Li C, Fu T, et al. Nanotechnology in therapeutics: A focus on nanoparticles as a drug delivery system. Nanomedicine. 2012;**7**:1253-1271. DOI: 10.2217/nnm.12.87

[24] Dobrovolskaia MA, Aggarwal P, Hall JB, McNeil SE. Preclinical studies to understand nanoparticle interaction with the immune system and its potential effects on nanoparticle biodistribution. Molecular Pharmaceutics. 2008;**5**:487-495. DOI: 10.1021/mp800032f

[25] Rautio J, Kumpulainen H, Heimbach T, Oliyai R, Oh D, Järvinen T, et al. Prodrugs: Design and clinical applications. Nature Reviews Drug Discovery. 2008;**7**:255-270. DOI: 10.1038/nrd2468

[26] Urban F. Prediction of human pharmacokinetics—Gut-wall metabolism. Journal of Pharmacy and Pharmacology. 2007;**59**(10):1335-1343. DOI: 10.1211/jpp.59.10.0002

[27] Wacher VJ, Salphati L, Benet LZ. Active secretion and enterocytic drug metabolism barriers to drug absorption. Advanced Drug Delivery Reviews. 2001;**46**:89-102. DOI: 10.1016/s0169-409x(00)00126-5

[28] Rothfield L, Justice S, García-Lara J. Bacterial cell division. Annual Review of Genetics. 1999;**33**:423-448. DOI: 10.1146/annurev.genet.33.1.423

[29] Rowlett VW, Margolin W. The bacterial min system. Current Biology. 2013;**23**:R553-R556. DOI: 10.1016/j.cub.2013.05.024

[30] Rowlett VW, Margolin W. The min system and other nucleoid-independent regulators of Z ring positioning. Frontiers in Microbiology. 2015;**6**:478. DOI: 10.3389/fmicb.2015.00478

[31] Lutkenhaus J, Addinall SG. Bacterial cell division and the Z ring. Annual Review of Biochemistry. 1997;**66**:93-116. DOI: 10.1146/annurev.biochem.66.1.93

[32] Adler HI, Fisher WD, Cohen A, Hardigree AA. Miniature *Escherichia coli* cells deficient in DNA. National Academy of Sciences of the United States of America. 1967;**57**:321-326. DOI: 10.1073/pnas.57.2.321

[33] Reeve JN, Mendelson NH, Coyne SI, Hallock LL, Cole RM. Minicells of *Bacillus subtilis*. Journal of Bacteriology. 1973;**114**(2):860-873. DOI: 10.1128/jb.114.2.860-873.1973

[34] Doan TTV, Nguyen HKT. Study on minicell generation of lactobacillus acidophilus VTCC-B-871 for drug delivery. Journal of Applied Pharmaceutical Science. 2013;**3**:33-36. DOI: 10.7324/JAPS.2013.3507

[35] Nguyen TH, Doan VT, Ha LD, Nguyen HN. Molecular cloning, expression of minD gene from *lactobacillus acidophilus* VTCC-B-871 and analyses to identify *lactobacillus rhamnosus* PN04 from Vietnam *Hottuynia cordata* Thunb. Indian Journal of Microbiology. 2013;**53**(4):385-390. DOI: 10.1007/s12088-013-0384-1

[36] Schär-Zammaretti P, Ubbink J. The cell wall of lactic acid bacteria: Surface constituents and macromolecular conformations. Biophysical Journal. 2003;**85**:4076-4092. DOI: 10.1016/S0006-3495(03)74820-6

[37] MacDiarmid JI, Amaro-Mugridge NB, Madrid-Weiss J, Sedliarou I, Wetzel S, Kochar K, et al. Sequential treatment of drug-resistant tumors with targeted minicells containing siRNA or a cytotoxic drug. Nature Biotechnology. 2009;**27**:643-651. DOI: 10.1038/nbt.1547

[38] Flemming A. Minicells deliver lethal load to tumours. Nature Reviews Drug Discovery. 2007;**6**:519-519. DOI: 10.1038/nrd2366

[39] Solomon BJ, Desai J, Rosenthal M, McArthur GA, Pattison ST, Pattison SL, et al. A first-time-In-human phase I clinical trial of bispecific antibody-targeted, paclitaxel-packaged bacterial minicells. PLoS One. 2015;**10**:e0144559. DOI: 10.1371/journal.pone.0144559

[40] Whittle JR, Lickliter JD, Gan HK, Scott AM, Simes J, Solomon BJ, et al. First in human nanotechnology doxorubicin delivery system to target epidermal growth factor receptors in recurrent glioblastoma. Journal of Clinical Neuroscience. 2015;**22**(12):1889-1894. DOI: 10.1016/j.jocn.2015.06.005

[41] Nguyen HN, Romero Jovel S, Nguyen THK. Nanosized Minicells generated by lactic acid bacteria for drug delivery. Journal of Nanomaterials. 2017;**2017**:1-10. DOI: 10.1155/2017/6847297

[42] Anggraeni VJ, Purwaniati P, Budiana W, Nurdin T. Molecular docking compounds in methanol extract of mango leaves (Mangifera indica L.) as anti-inflammatory agent. Jurnal Kimia Riset. 2022;7:57-65. DOI: 10.20473/jkr.v7i1.35950

[43] Ayipo YO, Yahaya SN, Babamale HF, Ahmad I, Patel H, Mordi MN. βCarboline alkaloids induce structural plasticity and inhibition of SARSCoV-2 nsp3 macrodomain more potently than remdesivir metabolite GS441524:

Computational approach. Turkish Journal of Biology. 2021;**45**:503-517. DOI: 10.3906/biy-2106-64

[44] Bandgar BP, Gawande SS. Synthesis and biological screening of a combinatorial library of β-chlorovinyl chalcones as anticancer, antiinflammatory and antimicrobial agents. Bioorganic & Medicinal Chemistry. 2010;**18**(5):2060-2065. DOI: 10.1016/j.bmc.2009.12.077

[45] Gurung AB, Bhattacharjee A, Ali MA. Exploring the physicochemical profile and the binding patterns of selected novel anticancer Himalayan plant derived active compounds with macromolecular targets. Informatics in Medicine Unlocked. 2016;**5**:1-14. DOI: 10.1016/j.imu.2016.09.004

[46] Nguyen KL, Nguyen HKT. Screening for potential anti-Alzheimer's compounds from *Angelica sinensis* extractions. World Journal of Pharmacy and Pharmaceutical Sciences. 2023;**12**(5):1347-1388. DOI: 10.20959/wjpps20235-24679